Keto Meal Prep

A Complete Guide for Beginners:

100+ Keto Meal Prep Recipes for Weight Loss, Fat Burning and Healthy Living.

Sarah Maddington © 2018

About Sarah Maddington

Sarah Maddington was born and raised in Manchester, UK. She is a Weight-Loss coach, Dietitian, Professional Chef and a mother of two. After finishing high school, she moved to London to pursue her dreams to study culinary.

In the past, Sarah was very overweight and suffered many health problems. She struggled with weight issues and found it difficult to maintain the balance between her career and her health.

It wasn't until after giving birth to her eldest daughter Sally, did she realise that she had to take her health more seriously if she wanted to become a role model for her children.
She lost 57 pounds in 6 months. Today, she wants to inspire beautiful people around the world to take control of the health so they can get back the life they deserve.

Table of Contents

Introduction

In this book you're going to learn all about meal prepping, what you need to get started, and meal prepping tips and tricks so that your meal prepping is successful. There are recipes here for everyone, from breakfast to dessert, and even snacks in between, there's a little something for everyone in this meal prepping book. Just remember that you'll want to take at least one day a week to dedicate to meal prepping so that you have enough food to last you through the week and free up your busy schedule. Just find the right recipes for you to get started.

Basics of Meal Prepping

Meal prepping is a technique that you use to lay out meals that you follow through the week, and this book focuses on ketogenic diet meals that can be prepped in advance. The object of meal prepping is to save both time and money.

Some Core Objectives

Here are some of main objectives of meal prepping.

- **Saving Money:** Meal prepping will help you to save money because it allows you to make a rough estimate of what you'll spend on food. You also know exactly what you need to buy and can look for the best bulk deals.
- **Sticking to Your Diet:** Meal prepping is used to help you to stick to a diet because you have three healthy meals a day planned and cooked in advance.
- **Minimize Waste:** By prepping your meals in advance, less food will spoil. You'll know exactly what you have, have it portioned out, and you'll even have a plan to eat it before it goes bad.
- **Limits Stress:** It helps to limit stress because you're no longer wandering what you should cook next.
- **Keeps Variety:** When you're meal prepping, you're going to have meals to choose from, which means it'll help you to keep variety in your routine.
- **Portion Control:** Meal prepping helps you to adjust to eating a certain amount of food per meal, which helps you to portion control. This is great on a diet because it really promotes weight loss by discouraging overeating.

- **Avoid Fast Food:** It helps you to avoid fast food because you're no longer having to make last minute preparations.
- **Frees Up Time:** While you'll be dedicating an entire day sometimes to meal prepping for the entire week, the rest of the weak you have more time because of it.

Kitchen Essentials

Below are some kitchen equipment essentials that you must have if you want to meal prep successfully.

- **Cutting Boards:** You're going to want to get a good cutting board if you're going to start preparing all of your meals yourself. Make sure to get them that are made out of solid materials such as marble, glass, rubber or plastic. They're corrosion resistant and they're non-porous. It helps make them easier to clean.
- **Measuring Cups:** It's going to take time away from what you should be doing if you're scrambling around for fades measuring cups. Make sure you have measuring cups that are clearly able to be read before starting.
- **Measuring Spoons:** Measuring spoons are often bought in sets, and you may want to invest in a new set before you start. You need to have all measurements easy to access before starting.
- **Non Metallic Containers:** Glass bowls will work perfectly for this. These are used to marinade, which won't change the properties or flavor of your food.
- **Packaging materials:** You're going to want fridge and freezer safe storage containers to pack your food away in. make sure they aren't metal so they can be microwave safe as well, and they should come

with a lid. This is also known as tin foil, and it's used to bake or even cover your food.

- **Aluminum Foil:**
- **Paper Towels & Kitchen Towels:** These help you to drain the meat.
- **Storage Space:** You're going to need cold storage space, so as long as you have a stand size fridge you should be fine. If you're really dedicated to meal prepping in advance, you may want to get a deep freezer as well.
- **Colander:** This is a bowl shaped utensil that has holes in it, allowing you to drain your food, including pasta and rice. You can also use it to rinse your vegetables.
- **Sharp Knives:** Most people only have dulled out knives in their kitchen, so invest in either new knives or a knife sharpener so that you can get started with ease.
- **Kitchen Scale:** This will help to make sure you're getting actuate measurements of condiments and meat.
- **Baking Sheet:** You'll want a flat, rectangular metal baking sheet so that you can make a lot of these recipes. They are also great to pop fat bombs into the freezer!
- **Internal Thermometer:** This will make sure that you get the right internal temperature with meats, including jerky, so you don't make yourself sick with these delightful homemade recipes.
- **Mesh Gloves:** These are for protection. Cutting meat will require precision and a sharp knife, so you'll want either butchering gloves, rubber gloves or mesh gloves to keep from getting hut when you're in a hurry.

About Storage Containers

Here are some tips about storage containers, which should help you to pick out practical and economical storage containers from stores near you. You can always check online for bulks deals too.

- **Glass:** For glass containers, you need to understand that they're great for long-term storage, but they are more expensive. They're heavier in weight too, so they're not the best ones to take on the go. However, they're easier to clean, and they're a great choice if you're worried about plastic safety or your carbon footprint.
- **Plastic:** These are lightweight and easy to carry, which is great if you eat on the go often. They're also convenient because you'll find them in a lot of different shapes and sizes, and they're easy to replace and dispose of.
- **Steel Containers:** These aren't what you'll want to heat your food in, but some people do get steel containers to avoid freezer burn.

Meal Prepping Tips

These tips and tricks will work better for some people than others, but it'll help you to get started with meal prepping.

Make a Plan

This is always recommended. If you don't have a plan, you're just going to end up cooking recipes that you pick at random, which could end up without any balance. You might cook too many dinner recipes and not enough breakfast recipes for the week, which would only leave you with stress and you'd have to cook later on in the week, defeating the purpose. It also helps to make sure you're eating the proper amount of net carbs if you've planned out your meals in advance. It's best to set a day aside to cook for at least seven days. If you're cooking enough meals, you'll probably have some carry over in to next week as well.

For the first time, you may need to cook for two days during that week to get enough meals up, but you'll slowly build up a stock in your freezer and fridge to help you get through the week. This helps to free up the rest of your week, but it only works wen everything is planned out in advance. By choosing your meals ahead of time, you're able to figure out how many portions you'll have to make sure you have enough, check the net carbs to make sure it's complying with your diet guidelines, and make sure you end up with enough variety that you feel comfortable meal prepping as a part of your routine.

Boil Eggs in the Oven

When you're using a pot, you sometimes can only boil five to six eggs, and your recipes might call for much more than that. If you're using your oven, then you're able to get out a muffin tin and boil twelve eggs at a time. Just put your eggs in the tin and then cover with water.

Put Your Smoothies in Bags

Freezer bags are great for smoothies because you can pop them out and into the blender again easily. Just add a little milk fi they're too thick or water if that's what you prefer using. They won't get stuck if you're using storage containers.

Use Skewers to Portion

When people think of skewers, they usually think of grilling kabobs, but this isn't always the case. You can skewer your meat even after cooking it so that you divide your meat evenly between containers. For example, out of a batch that makes four servings, you can get out eight skewers. Fill up the eight skewers with equal parts meat, and then put two skewers into each container so it's portioned out properly.

Pencil on the Date

You're going to want to make sure that you either put down the date the food goes bad by doing the math beforehand or at least the date on when you prepared the food on your containers. A lot of people take a pen and masking tape, writing it on the masking tape to put on their containers and just peeling it off when they do a new batch. You can get sick from eating old food, so you need to know how long everything will last in the fridge and freezer. As a general rule of thumb, after four to five days in the fridge something needs thrown out unless the recipe says otherwise. For the freezer, throw something out after a month or if it has freezer burn.

Keep Mason Jars

If you're preparing salads a lot for lunch, mason jars are a great way to keep them in the fridge. Just put the salad dressing at the bottom so that none of your greens go soggy, and you can mix it up before you eat. It allows you to layer everything so that you know exactly what you have in each jar too. You're going to want to keep seven to twelve jars on hand.

Breakfast Recipes

Breakfast recipes are an important part of the day, and it can be difficult to find time for it during a busy schedule. Luckily, with these recipes, keto friendly meal prepping recipes, it's a little easier.

#1 Breakfast Tapas

Serve: 6

Time: 5 Minutes

Calories: 749

Protein: 41 Grams

Fat: 58 Grams

Net Carbs: 15 Grams

Ingredients:

- 8 Ounces Mozzarella, Shredded
- 8 Ounces Gouda
- 8 Ounces Salami
- 8 Ounces Prosciutto
- 2 Cucumbers, Sliced
- 2 Bell Peppers, Sliced
- 2 Avocados, Pitted
- 4 Tablespoons Mayonnaise
- Black Pepper to Taste
- 2 Ounces Walnuts
- 2 Ounces Almonds

Directions:

1. Chop your cheese and meat into bite size pieces, spreading it across three plates, and then divide your cucumbers and peppers. Make sure to divide your nuts too.
2. In a bowl scoop the avocado from its skin, and then add in the bowl. Add in your mayonnaise and pepper. Mash well, and divide that among the plates too.

#2 Coconut Cream with Berries

Serves: 4

Time: 5 Minutes

Calories: 584

Protein: 13 Grams

Fat: 57 Grams

Net Carbs: 10 Grams

Ingredients:

- 1 Cup Berries, Frozen
- 16 Ounces Almonds
- 2 Cups Coconut Milk, Unsweet & Full Fat
- Cinnamon to Taste

Directions:

1. Whip your coconut milk until creamy using a mixer.
2. Spoon your coconut milk cream into bowls, topping with berries and almonds.
3. Sprinkle cinnamon on top before serving. You can keep this in the fridge.

#3 Blueberry Scones

Serves: 12

Time: 25 Minutes

Calories: 133

Protein: 2 Grams

Fat: 8 Grams

Net Crabs: 4 Grams

Ingredients:

- 3 Eggs, Large & Beaten
- ½ Cup Stevia
- 2 Teaspoon Vanilla Extract, Pure
- 2 Teaspoon Baking Powder
- 1 ½ Cups Almond Flour
- ¾ Cup Raspberries, Frozen

Directions:

1. Heat your oven to 375, and then line a baking sheet with parchment paper.
2. In a bowl mix your eggs, stevia, vanilla extract, almond flour, baking powder, and whisk well.
3. Fold in your raspberries, stirring until well combined.
4. Scoop the batter onto a baking sheet, making sure it's even mounds. Keep two inches between each mound, and then bake for fifteen minutes.
5. Bake for fifteen minutes, and allow to cool.

#4 Peanut Butter Cup Smoothie

Serves: 4

Time: 10 Minutes

Calories: 486

Protein: 30 Grams

Fat: 40 Grams

Net Carbs: 6 Grams

Ingredients:

- 2 Cups Water
- 2 Scoop Chocolate Protein Powder
- 1 ½ Cups Coconut Cream
- 6 Ice Cubes
- 4 Tablespoons Natural Peanut Butter

Directions:

1. Pour everything into a blender, and blend well until smooth.

#5 Tofu & Mushrooms

Serves: 6

Time: 30 Minutes

Calories: 211

Protein: 11.5 Grams

Fat: 18.5 Grams

Net Carbs: 1.6 Grams

Ingredients:

- 2 Cups Mushrooms, Fresh & Chopped Fine
- 8 Tablespoons Parmesan Cheese, Shredded
- 2 Blocks Tofu, Cubed into 1 Inch Pieces
- 8 Tablespoons Butter
- Sea Salt & Black Pepper to Taste

Directions:

1. Mix your salt, pepper and tofu together.
2. Get out a pan and heat your butter over medium-low heat.
3. Add in your tofu, cooking for five minutes.
4. Stir in your mushrooms and parmesan, cooking for another four minutes. Don't forget to stir so nothing sticks.

#6 Vegetable & Bacon Dish

Serves: 4

Time: 30 Minutes

Calories: 197

Protein: 14.3 Grams

Fat: 13.8 Grams

Net Carbs: 3.1 Grams

Ingredients:

- 1 Tablespoon Avocado Mayonnaise
- 2 Scallions, Chopped
- ½ Cup Parmesan Cheese
- 1 Green Bell Pepper, Seeded & Chopped
- 4 Bacon Slices

Directions:

1. Start by heating your oven to 375, and then grease a baking dish. Arrange the bacon in your baking dish with bell peppers on top. Add your mayonnaise and parmesan next, sprinkling with scallions.
2. Bake for twenty-five minutes.

#7 Tofu & Onion Scramble

Serves: 8

Time: 20 Minutes

Calories: 184

Protein: 12.2 Grams

Fat: 12.7 Grams

Net Carbs: 4.7 Grams

Ingredients:

- 4 Onions, Sliced
- 8 Tablespoons Butter
- 2 Cups Cheddar Cheese, Grated
- 4 Blocks Tofu, Pressed & Cubed into 1 Inch Pieces
- Sea Salt & Black Pepper to Taste

Directions:

1. Start by seasoning your tofu with salt and pepper, and then butter your pan.
2. Place your pan over medium-low heat, adding in your tofu.
3. Add your onions in next, and cook for three minutes.
4. Add in your tofu next, cooking for another two minutes.
5. Add in the cheese, and cover with a lid, cooking for five more minutes.

#8 Bok Choy Samba

Serves: 6

Time: 20 Minutes

Calories: 112

Protein: 3 Grams

Fat: 4.9 Grams

Net Carbs: 1.5 Grams

Ingredients:

- 8 Tablespoons Cream
- 2 Tablespoons Olive Oil
- 4 Bacon Slices
- 8 Bok Choy Slices
- 1 Cup Parmesan Cheese, Grated
- Sea Salt & Black Pepper to Taste

Directions:

1. Sprinkle your bok choy with salt and pepper, and oil your skillet.
2. Place your skillet over medium-high heat, and then add in your bacon. Cook for five minutes, and then stir in your cream and bok choy. Cook for six minutes.
3. Top with parmesan and cook for another four minutes over low heat.

#9 English Breakfast

Serves: 4

Time: 25 Minutes

Calories: 404

Protein: 17 Grams

Fat: 34 Grams

Net Carbs: 3 Grams

Ingredients:

- 4 Eggs, Large
- 2 Avocados, Sliced
- 2 Cups Mushrooms, Sliced
- 4 Sausage Links
- 8 Bacon Slices, Uncured
- Sea Salt & Black Pepper to Taste

Directions:

1. Scramble your eggs before placing them to the side. Put your bacon and sausage in the skillet, cooking until browned, which should take eight to ten minutes. Drain them on a paper towel lined plate.
2. Add in your mushrooms to the pan, and cook for five to six minutes. Make sure to stir frequently to keep them from burning. They should be browned and softened.
3. Arrange everything on a plate, and allow it to cool before freezing.

#10 Green Berry Smoothie

Serves: 4

Time: 20 Minutes

Calories: 436

Protein: 28 Grams

Fat: 36 Grams

Net Carbs: 6 Grams

Ingredients:

- 2 Cup Water
- 1 Cup Raspberries
- 1 Cup Kale, Shredded
- 2 Tablespoon Coconut Oil
- 1 ½ Cup Cream Cheese
- 2 Scoop Vanilla Protein Powder

Directions:

1. Put everything into a blender and blend until smooth.

Lemon & Lavender Ricotta Pancakes

Serves: 4

Time: 25 Minutes

Calories: 279

Protein: 18 Grams

Fat: 20 Grams

Net Carbs: 2 Grams

Ingredients:

- 8 Egg, Large
- ½ Cup Ricotta Cheese
- 4 Teaspoons Vanilla Bean Sweetener
- 2 Teaspoon Lemon Juice, Fresh
- 4 Tablespoons Coconut Flour
- 2 Tablespoons Culinary Lavender
- 1 Teaspoon Baking Powder
- 2 Tablespoons Golden Ghee
- 2 Lemons, Zested
- Grass Fed Butter
- Maple Syrup, Sugar Free

Directions:

1. Blend your eggs, ricotta cheese, lemon juice, lavender, coconut flour, sweetener and baking powder together. Just blend on low for ten seconds.
2. Melt your ghee over medium heat in a skillet, and then pour a quarter cup of your batter in the center, and then cook until the bottom is crispy and brown. This should take a minute. Flip your pancake over and brown on the other side for about a minute more. continue to cook until you run out of batter
3. Sprinkle with lemon zest and maple syrup before serving. When freezing, do not add your maple syrup first.

#11 Blueberry Spinach Smoothie

Serves: 4

Time: 5 Minutes

Calories: 353

Protein: 15 Grams

Fat: 32 Grams

Net Carbs: 6 Grams

Ingredients:

- 2 Cup Coconut Milk
- 2 Cup Spinach
- 1 Cup Blueberries
- 1 English Cucumber, Chopped
- 2 Scoop Protein Powder
- 4 Tablespoons Coconut Oil
- Mint Sprigs For Garnish
- 8 Ice Cubes

Directions:

1. Blend everything together until smooth.

#12 Cajun Egg Hash

Serves: 4

Time: 30 Minutes

Calories: 260

Protein: 22 Grams

Fat: 15 Grams

Net Carbs: 6 Grams

Ingredients:

- ½ Green Bell Pepper, Chopped
- 8 Ounces Pastrami, Shaved & Chopped
- 4 Eggs, Large & Beaten
- ½ Sweet Yellow Onion, Chopped
- ½ Green Bell Pepper, Chopped
- 2 Tablespoon Garlic, Minced
- 1 Teaspoon Cajun Seasoning

Directions:

1. Put your steamer basket inside of a pot, and then pour enough after to cover he bottom of the pot. Bring your water to a boil using high eat, and then add in your cauliflower. Cover the pot, and steam it until your cauliflower is tender. This should take about six minutes.
2. Drain it, and chop it into bite size pieces before setting it to the side.
3. In a medium skillet, heat your oil using medium heat, and then add in your onion. Sauté until it gets soft, but do not brown it. This should take three to five minutes.

4. Put your eggs in a skillet, scrambling them with your onion for two minutes.

5. Add in your remaining ingredients, and cook for five minutes more.

#13 Cinnamon Smoothie

Serves: 4

Time: 5 Minutes

Calories: 492

Protein: 18 Grams

Fat: 47 Grams

Net Carbs: 6 Grams

Ingredients:

- 2 Teaspoons Cinnamon
- 1 Teaspoon Vanilla Extract, Pure
- 10 Drops Liquid Stevia
- 4 Cups Coconut Milk
- 1 Scoop Vanilla Protein Powder

Directions:

1. Blend everything together until smooth.

#14 Mushrooms Frittata

Serves: 6

Time: 25 Minutes

Calories: 316

Protein: 16 Grams

Fat: 27 Grams

Net Carbs: 1 Grams

Ingredients:

- 1/2 Cup Goat Cheese, Crumbled
- 2 Tablespoons Olive oil
- 1 Cup Mushrooms, Fresh & Sliced
- 1 Cup Spinach, Shredded
- 6 Bacon Slices, Cooked & Chopped
- 10 Eggs, Large & Beaten
- Sea Salt & Black Pepper to Taste

Directions:

1. Start by preheating your oven to 350.
2. Get out an ovenproof skillet, and then put it over medium-high heat. Add in your olive oil to heat it up.
3. Once it's heated up, sauté the mushrooms for three minutes. They should be browned lightly.
4. Add your bacon, spinach and sauté until your spinach wilts. This should take about a minute.
5. Add your eggs lifting so they flow underneath. Cook for three to four minutes.

6. Sprinkle your goat cheese on top before seasoning with salt and
   pepper.

7. Bake until browned, which should set for fifteen minutes.

8. Allow it to stand for five minutes before cutting it into six wedges.

#15 Cream Cheese & Cinnamon Eggs

Serves: 6

Time: 20 Minutes

Calories: 119

Protein: 4 Grams

Fat: 11 Grams

Net Carbs: 1 Gram

Ingredients:

- 6 Tablespoons Cream Cheese, Room Temperature
- 2 Tablespoons Heavy Whipping Cream
- 3 Eggs, Large
- ½ Teaspoon Cinnamon
- 1 Teaspoons Coconut Flour
- 1 Tablespoon Golden Ghee
- Sweetener to Taste

Directions:

1. Combine your cream cheese, heavy cream, coconut flour, cinnamon, eggs and sweetener in a blender, blending well.
2. Get out a medium skillet and place it over medium heat. Melt your ghee before adding in your cream cheese and egg mixture.
3. Scramble and cook all the way through, which should take about five minutes.

#16 Avocado & Basil Smoothie

Serves: 4

Time: 5 Minutes

Calories: 343

Protein: 25 Grams

Fat: 22 Grams

Net Carbs: 4 Grams

Ingredients:

- 4 Cups Almond Milk, Unsweetened
- 8 Ice Cubes
- 4 Tablespoons Basil, Fresh & Chopped
- 2 Teaspoons Ginger, Grated
- 1 1/3 Cup Vanilla Whey Protein Powder, Low Carb
- 2 Avocados, Chopped

Directions:

1. Blend everything together until it's smooth. Section out before freezing.

#17 Rosemary Quiche

Serves: 6

Time: 40 Minutes

Calories: 184

Protein: 12 Grams

Fat: 14 Grams

Net Carbs: 1 Gram

Ingredients:

- ½ Cup Heavy Whipping Cream
- 6 Eggs, Large
- 1 Teaspoon Rosemary Infused Olive Oil
- 2 Tablespoons Cream Cheese, Room Temperature
- 7 Ounces Ham, Cubed
- 1 Teaspoon Sea Salt, Fine
- 1 Teaspoon Rosemary, Fresh & Chopped

Directions:

1. Start by preheating your oven to 375, and then get out a nine inch pie dish. Rub it down with your rosemary olive oil.
2. Get out a bowl and beat your eggs lightly, stirring in your ham, rosemary, cream cheese, salt and heavy cream. Make sure it's mixed well.
3. Pour your egg mixture into your pie dish, baking until the eggs are set and golden brown. This will take about a half hour.
4. Allow it to sit for ten minutes before slicing.

#18 Strawberry Sage Smoothie

Serves: 4

Time: 5 Minutes

Calories: 173

Protein: 2 Grams

Fat: 16 Grams

Net Carbs: 5 Grams

Ingredients:

- 4 Cups Coconut Milk, Unsweetened
- 4 Sage Leaves, Fresh
- 20 Strawberries, Frozen
- 8 Tablespoons Heavy Whipping Cream
- 4 Teaspoons Vanilla Bean Sweetener, Sugar Free

Directions:

1. Blend everything together until smooth, and then section out into serving cups before freezing.

#19 Breakfast Meatloaf

Serves: 4

Time: 45 Minutes

Calories: 682

Protein: 38 Grams

Fat: 24 Grams

Net Carbs: 4.5 Grams

Ingredients:

- 6 Eggs, Large
- Golden Ghee
- 1 lb. Bulk Sausage
- ¼ Yellow Onion, Chopped
- 4 Ounces Cream Cheese, Room Temperature & Divided
- 2 Tablespoons Scallions, Chopped
- 1 Cup Cheddar Cheese, Shredded

Directions:

1. Start by heating your oven to 350, and then grease a loaf pan with your ghee.
2. Beat your eggs in a bowl, and then add in your onion and sausage. Add in half of your cream cheese, and mix well.
3. Pour your egg and meatloaf mixtures into the loaf pan, and then bake uncovered for a half hour.
4. Remove it from the oven and allow it to sit for five minutes.

5. Scrape off the excess fat from the top, and then top with the remaining cream cheese and cheddar cheese. Sprinkle your scallions over it.

6. Bake for another five minutes, and then broil for three more minutes.

7. Allow it to sit for five minutes before slicing.

#20 Frozen Coffee Delight

Serves: 2

Time: 5 Minutes

Calories: 488

Protein: 3 Grams

Fat: 52 Grams

Net Carbs: 0 Grams

Ingredients:

- 1 Cup Whipped Cream
- 14 Ice Cubes
- 2 Cups Cold Brew Coffee
- 2/3 Heavy Whipping Cream
- 4 Tablespoons Vanilla Bean Sweetener, Sugar Free

Directions:

1. Blend everything together, and then pour into serving cups before freezing.

Lunch Recipes

You won't want to always freeze your lunches, but these ketogenic recipes do keep in the fridge to help make your week a little easier.

#21 Egg Drop Soup

Serves: 4

Time: 289

Protein: 15.3 Grams

Fat: 23.24 Grams

Net Carbs: 2.92 Grams

Ingredients:

- 4 Teaspoons Chili Garlic Paste
- 8 Eggs, Large
- 2 Chicken Bouillon Cubes
- 4 Tablespoons Bacon Fat
- 6 Cups Chicken Broth

Directions:

1. Put a pan over medium high heat, and add in your chicken broth, bacon fat and bouillon cubes.
2. Bring it to a boil and then add in your chili garlic paste. Make sure to stir well, and then turn off the heat.
3. Beat your eggs, pouring it into your broth.
4. Stir well, and allow it to settle.

#22 Cashew Chicken

Serves: 3

Time: 25 Minutes

Calories: 333

Protein: 22.6 Grams

Fat: 24 Grams

Net Carbs: 6.7 Grams

Ingredients:

- ¼ Cup Cashews, Raw
- 2 Tablespoons Coconut Oil
- ¼ Cup Cashews, Raw
- 3 Chicken Thighs, Boneless & Skinless
- ½ Green Bell Pepper, Sliced
- ½ Teaspoon Ginger
- 1 Tablespoon Rice Wine Vinegar
- 1 ½ Tablespoons Liquid Aminos
- ½ Tablespoon Chili Garlic Sauce
- 1 Tablespoon Sesame Oil
- 1 Tablespoon Garlic, Minced
- 1 Tablespoon Sesame Seeds
- 1 Tablespoon Green Onions, Sliced
- ¼ White Onion, Medium
- Sea Salt & Black Pepper to Taste

Directions:

1. Put a pan over low heat, and then toast your cashews, cooking for
   eight minutes. They should burn brown lightly, and they should
   become fragrant. Place them to the side.
2. Dice your chicken thighs, cubing them into one inch chunks, cutting up
   your onion and pepper as well.
3. Place your pan over high heat, adding in your coconut toil.
4. Add in your chicken meat, and then let them cook all the way through.
   This should take five minutes.
5. Once your chicken has cooked, add in your onion and green bell
   pepper. Toss with chili garlic sauté, ginger, salt, pepper and garlic.
   Cook for two to three minutes.
6. Add in your rice wine vinegar, cashews and liquid aminos, cooking on
   high until the liquid reduces. It should have a sticky consistency, and
   then serve with sesame seeds and drizzled with sesame oil.

#23 Broccoli & Cauliflower Salad

Serves: 7

Time: 15 Minutes

Calories: 324

Protein: 7 Grams

Fat: 32Grams

Net Carbs: 3 Grams

Ingredients:

- 8 Ounces Broccoli Florets Chopped
- 8 Ounces Cauliflower Florets, Chopped
- 4 Ounces Cheddar Cheese, Diced
- 2 Ounces Red Pepper, Diced
- 1/3 lbs. Bacon, Cooked & Crumbled
- 2 Tablespoons Red Onion, Chopped
- ¾ Cup Mayonnaise
- ¾ Cup Greek Yogurt, Plain
- 2 Tablespoons Swerve
- 1 Tablespoon Lemon Juice, Fresh

Directions:

1. Start by combining your cauliflower, red pepper, cheese, onion and broccoli together.
2. Get out a bowl, and stir together your yogurt, mayonnaise, swerve and lemon juice. Adjust to taste.
3. Toss all of your ingredients together.

#24 Garlic Soup

Serves: 10

Time: 1 Hour 10 Minutes

Calories: 142

Protein: 4.1 Grams

Fat: 8.4 Grams

Net Carbs: 2.6 Grams

Ingredients:

- 1 Tablespoon Olive Oil
- 2 Bulbs Garlic, Peeled
- 3 Shallots, Chopped
- 1 Large Cauliflower, Chopped
- 6 Cups Vegetable Broth
- Sea Salt & Black Pepper to Taste

Directions:

1. Start by heating your oven to 400. Slice ¼ inch off the top of your garlic bulbs, and then wrap it in aluminum foil. Grease with olive oil, roasting for thirty-five minutes.
2. Squeeze the flesh from your roasted garlic. Heat your oil in a saucepan, and then add in your shallots. Cook for six minutes, and then add in your garlic. Toss in your remaining ingredients.
3. Reduce the heat to low and cover the pan.
4. Allow it to cook fifteen to twenty minutes. Puree the mixture, and season with salt and pepper before serving.

#25 Goat Cheese Salad

Serves: 4

Time: 45 Minutes

Calories: 474

Protein: 24.5 Grams

Fat: 40.8 Grams

Net Carbs: 3.1 Grams

Ingredients:

- 10 Ounces Goat Cheese, Sliced
- 4 Tablespoons Pumpkin Seeds
- 1 Tablespoon Balsamic Vinegar
- 2 Ounces Butter
- 3 Ounces Baby Spinach

Directions:

1. Start by heating your oven to 400.
2. Spread your cheese on a baking dish, baking for ten minutes.
3. Put your pumpkin seeds into a skillet, and roast until thy change color, and then reduce the heat. Add butter, and allow it to simmer until they turn golden.
4. Add vinegar, bringing the mixture to a boil, and then turn off the heat. Stir in your spinach, and allow it to rest for five minutes before transferring to a serving dish. Top with cheese before serving.

#26 Eggplant Salad

Serves: 3

Time: 40 Minutes

Calories: 196

Protein: 14.3 Grams

Fat: 10.4 Grams

Net Carbs: 12.6 Grams

Ingredients:

- 2 Eggplant, Peeled & Sliced
- 2 Greens Bell Peppers, Sliced & Seeded
- ½ Cup Parsley, Fresh
- ½ Cup Mayonnaise
- 2 Cloves Garlic
- Sea Salt & Black Pepper to Taste

Directions:

1. Heat your oven to 480, and then add in your eggplants and bell pepper into a baking dish, baking for a half hour. Flip your vegetables after twenty minutes, and then add all of your ingredients into a bowl.
2. Mix well before serving.

#27 Creamy Leeks

Serves: 6

Time: 35 Minutes

Calories: 204

Protein: 6.3 Grams

Fat: 15.7 Grams

Net Carbs: 11.5 Grams

Ingredients:

- 2 Ounces butter
- 1 ½ lbs. Leeks, Trimmed & Chopped into 4 Inch Pieces
- 1 Cup Coconut Cream
- Sea Salt & Black Pepper to Taste
- 3 ½ Ounces Cheddar Cheese

Directions:

1. Start by heating your oven to 400, and then place your butter in a skillet.
2. Place your skillet over medium heat, and add in your leeks.
3. Sauté for five minutes, and then put them in a greased baking dish.
4. Boil your cream in a saucepan over low heat, and then stir in your cheese. Season with salt and pepper, and then pour this over the leeks.
5. Bake for fifteen to twenty minutes.

#28 Chicken Tenders

Serves: 6

Time: 25 Minutes

Calories: 447

Protein: 47.7 Grams

Fat: 26.4 Grams

Net Carbs: 2.3 Grams

Ingredients:

- 1 Cup Cream
- 4 Tablespoons Butter
- 1 Cup Feta Cheese
- 2 lbs. Chicken Tenders
- Sea Salt & Black Pepper to Taste

Directions:

1. Start by heating your oven to 350, and then grease your baking dish with cooking spray.
2. Sprinkle your chicken tenders with salt and pepper before setting it to the side for ten minutes.
3. Heat up your butter in a pan, and then add the chicken tenders. Cook for five minutes per side, and then top with cream and feta cheese, baking for fifteen minutes.

#29 Salmon Stew

Serves: 6

Time: 20 Minutes

Calories: 272

Protein: 32.1 Grams

Fat: 14.2 Grams

Net Carbs: 3.3 Grams

Ingredients:

- 2 Onions, Chopped
- 2 Cups Fish Broth
- 2 lbs. Salmon Fillet, Cubed
- 2 Tablespoons Butter
- Sea Salt & Black Pepper to Taste

Directions:

1. Season the fillet with salt and pepper, and then heat your butter in a skillet. Add in your onions, cooking for three minutes.
2. Add in your salmon, cooking for two minutes per side.
3. Add in your fish broth, cooking for seven minutes while covered.

#30 Vegetable Bacon Soup

Serves: 4

Time: 20 Minutes

Calories: 424

Protein: 26.6 Grams

Fat: 31.4 Grams

Net Carbs: 6.5 Grams

Ingredients:

- 6 Turkey Bacon Slices, Cooked & Chopped
- 1 Head Cauliflower, Chopped Roughly
- 2 Cups Cheddar Cheese, Shredded
- 1 Tablespoon Olive Oil
- 4 Dashes Hot Pepper Sauce
- 1 Cup Half & Half
- 1 Yellow Onion, Chopped
- 2 Cloves Garlic, Minced
- 4 Cups Chicken Broth
- Black Pepper to Taste

Directions:

1. Place your olive oil in a pot, and then add in your onion and garlic. Cook for three minutes before adding your broth and cauliflower. Season with salt and pepper.
2. Cover the lid, and cook for twenty minutes over medium-low heat.
3. Open the lid to add your remaining ingredients, cooking for five more minutes.

#31 Spinach Quiche

Serves: 6

Time: 45 Minutes

Calories: 349

Protein: 23 Grams

Fat: 27.8 Grams

Net Carbs: 1.9 Grams

Ingredients:

- 10 Ounces Frozen Spinach, Thawed
- 5 Eggs, Beaten
- 1 Tablespoons Butter, Melted
- 3 Cups Monterrey Jack Cheese, Shredded
- Sea Salt & Black Pepper to Taste

Directions:

1. Start by heating your oven to 350, and then grease a nine in pie dish.
2. Place your butter in a skillet, placing it over medium-low heat, and then add in your spinach. Cook for three minutes before setting it aside.
3. Mix your eggs, cheese and spinach together, seasoning it with salt and pepper.
4. Put the mixture into a pie dish, and then cook for another half hour.
5. Allow it to cool before slicing.

#32 Cheese Casserole

Serves: 6

Time: 40 Minutes

Calories: 521

Protein: 35.4 Grams

Fat: 38.8 Grams

Net Carbs: 6 Grams

Ingredients:

- 10 Ounce Parmesan, Shredded
- 16 Ounces Mozzarella, Shredded
- 2 lbs. Sausage, Scrambled
- 2 Tablespoons Olive oil
- 16 Ounces Marinara Sauce

Directions:

1. Start by heating the oven to 375, and then grease a baking dish using your olive oil.
2. Put half o your sausage scramble in your baking dish, and then spread your marinara over it. Top with your mozzarella and parmesan next, and then put the remaining sausage over it, and then top with the remaining parmesan and mozzarella, drizzling more marinara over it.
3. Bake for twenty to twenty-two minutes.

#33 Cheddar & Cauliflower Soup

Serves: 8

Time: 40 Minutes

Calories: 227

Protein: 8 Grams

Fat: 21 Grams

Net Carbs: 2 Grams

Ingredients:

- 1 Head Cauliflower, Chopped
- ½ Sweet Onion, Chopped
- ¼ Cup Butter
- 4 Cups Herbed Chicken Stock
- 1 Cup Heavy Whipping Cream
- ½ Teaspoon Nutmeg
- 1 Cup Cheddar Cheese, Shredded
- Sea Salt & Black Pepper to Taste

Directions:

1. Get out a large stockpot and place your butter in it before putting it over medium heat.
2. Sauté your cauliflower and onion until it's lightly browned and tender. It should take about ten minutes.
3. Add in your nutmeg and chicken stock, bringing it to a boil.
4. Reduce the heat to low, and allow it to simmer until your vegetables are tender. This should take about fifteen minutes.

5. Remove it from heat, stirring in your cream. Puree with an immersion blender, and then season with salt and pepper. Top with cheddar cheese before serving.

#34 Tomato Soup

Serves: 8

Time: 30 Minutes

Calories: 194

Protein: 9.2 Grams

Fat: 15.4 Grams

Net Carbs: 4.2 Grams

Ingredients:

- 2 Teaspoons Basil, Crushed
- 4 Cups Vegetable Broth, Low Sodium
- 4 Tablespoon Erythritol
- 1 Tablespoon Balsamic Vinegar
- ½ Cup Basil, Fresh & Chopped
- 1 Tablespoon Olive Oil
- 2 Cloves Garlic, Minced
- 2 lbs. Tomatoes, Fresh & Chopped
- 2 Teaspoons Parsley
- 2 Cups Cheddar Cheese
- Black Pepper to Taste

Directions:

1. Place your tomatoes garlic, herbs, broth and black pepper into a pot with your oil.
2. Cover, and cook for twenty minutes over medium-low heat.
3. Stir in your vinegar and sugar, and then use an immersion blender to blend your soup.

4. Garnish with basil before serving.

#35 BLT Salad

Serves: 4

Time: 15 Minutes

Calories: 228

Protein: 1 Gram

Fat: 18 Grams

Net Carbs: 2 Grams

Ingredients:

- 2 Tablespoons Bacon Fat, Melted
- 2 Tablespoons Red Wine Vinegar
- 4 Cups Lettuce, shredded
- Black Pepper to Taste
- 1 Tomato, Chopped
- 6 Bacon Slices, Cooked & Chopped
- 2 Eggs, Hardboiled & Chopped
- 1 Tablespoons Sunflower Seeds, Roasted & Unsalted
- 1 Teaspoon Sesame Seeds, Toasted
- 1 Chicken, Cooked & Sliced

Directions:

1. Whisk together your vinegar and bacon fat until it emulsifies. Season with pepper, and then add your tomato and lettuce in a bowl.
2. Toss your vegetables with the dressing, dividing your salad between plates.
3. Top with bacon, sunflower seeds, sesame seeds, egg and chicken. Keep the dressing separate until you're ready to serve.

#36 Avocado Egg Salad

Serves: 4

Time: 5 Minutes

Calories: 259

Protein: 11 Grams

Fat: 21 Grams

Net Carbs: 4 Grams

Ingredients:

- 6 Eggs, Hardboiled
- 2 Avocados, Pitted & Divided
- 1 Teaspoon Mustard
- 1 Tablespoon Lemon Juice, Fresh
- 1 Tablespoon Apple Cider Vinegar
- 1 Teaspoon Garlic Powder
- ½ Teaspoon Paprika
- Sea Salt & Black Pepper to Taste
- Romaine Lettuce for Serving

Directions:

1. Mash one avocado and three of your eggs with your mustard, vinegar, lemon juice, garlic and paprika in a bowl.
2. Chop the other egg yolks and whites, adding them to the avocado mixture.
3. Dice the avocado, and stir it into the mixture. Make sure to season it with salt and pepper, serving on your romaine leaves.

#37 Avocado & Chicken Wraps

Serves: 4

Time: 10 Minutes

Calories: 264

Protein: 12 Grams

Fat: 20 Grams

Net Carbs: 6 Grams

Ingredients:

- ½ Avocado, Peeled & Pitted
- 1 Teaspoon Lemon Juice, Fresh
- 1/3 Cup Creamy Mayonnaise
- 2 Teaspoons Thyme Leaves, Fresh & Chopped
- 6 Ounces Chicken Breast, Cooked & Chopped
- 8 Large Lettuce Leaves for Serving
- ¼ Cup Walnuts, Chopped
- Sea Salt & Black Pepper to Taste

Directions:

1. Mash your avocados in a bowl, and ten add in your thyme, mayonnaise and lemon juice.
2. Stir in your chicken, seasoning with salt and pepper.
3. Keep your lettuce leaves and walnuts separate until you're ready to serve.

#38 Sausage & Shrimp Bake

Serves: 4

Time: 35 Minutes

Calories: 323

Protein: 20 Grams

Fat: 24 Grams

Net Carbs: 6 Grams

Ingredients:

- 2 Tablespoons olive oil
- 6 Ounces Chorizo Sausage, Diced
- 1 Red Bell Pepper, Chopped
- ½ lb. Shrimp, Peeled & Deveined
- ½ Small Sweet Onion, Chopped
- 2 Teaspoons Garlic, Minced
- ¼ Cup Herbed Chicken Stock
- Pinch Red Pepper Flakes

Directions:

1. Put a skillet over medium-high heat and then add in your olive oil.
2. Sauté your sausage, warming it all the way through for six minutes.
3. Add in your shrimp, and cook until it turns opaque. This should take four minutes.
4. Remove your sausage and shrimp, placing it in a bowl.
5. Place your onion, garlic and red pepper in your skillet, cooking for four minutes or until your vegetables are tender.

6. Add in your chicken's tock, and then add your sausage and shrimp back in.

7. Bring it to a simmer, cooking for three minutes.

8. Stir in your red pepper flakes before taking it off the stove and allowing it to cool.

#39 Pumpkin Curry Chicken

Serves: 4

Time: 25 Minutes

Calories: 540

Protein: 54 Grams

Fat: 32 Grams

Net Carbs: 7 Grams

Ingredients:

- 14 Ounces Pumpkin Puree, Pure
- 1 Cup Coconut Milk, Unsweetened
- 4 Tablespoons Ghee
- 2 Tablespoons Lime Juice, Fresh
- 1 Small White Onion, Chopped
- 4 Tablespoon Thai Basil Leaves, Chopped & Fresh
- 2 Teaspoons Curry Powder
- 1 Teaspoon Coriander
- 1 Teaspoon Cinnamon
- 1 Teaspoon Ginger
- 1 Teaspoon Sea Salt + More for Seasoning
- 1 Teaspoon Red Pepper Flakes
- 4 Tablespoons Olive Oil
- 2 lbs. Chicken Tenders
- Black Pepper to Taste

Directions:

1. Blend your pumpkin, coconut milk, lime juice, onion, ghee, Thai basil, curry powder, cinnamon, ginger, coriander, slat and red pepper flakes in a blender.

2. Get out a small saucepan, and pour in the mixture, placing it over medium heat.

3. In another skillet, heat your olive oil, and season your chicken tenders using salt and pepper. Once your oil is shimmering, add in your chicken tenders. Cook three minutes per side, and then chop it into one inch pieces, adding it into your pumpkin curry. Reduce your heat to low, cooking for five to ten minutes more so it's heated all the way through.

#40 Burrata Caprese Salad

Serves: 4

Time: 5 Minutes

Calories: 188

Protein: 4 Grams

Net Carbs: 3 Grams

Ingredients:

- 10 Basil Leaves, Fresh
- 2 Tomatoes
- Sea Salt to Taste
- Black Pepper to Taste
- 8 Ounce Burrata Cheese Ball
- Olive Oil to Taste

Directions:

1. Star by slicing your tomatoes, and put them on a plate. Sprinkle with salt, and then add in your basil leaves. Sprinkle with more salt, and then slice your cheese ball.
2. Add it on top of your plate, and season with olive oil and pepper. Section out before refrigerating.

#41 Creamy Kale & Sausage Soup

Serves: 6

Time: 30 Minutes

Calories: 470

Protein: 4 Grams

Fat: 45 Grams

Net Carbs: 3 Grams

Ingredients:

- ½ Cup Pancetta
- ½ Cup Onion, Chopped
- 1 lb. Italian Bulk Sausage
- 2 Cups Kale, Chopped
- Sea Salt to Taste
- ½ Teaspoon Italian Seasoning
- ½ Teaspoon Black Pepper
- 1 Tablespoon Garlic, Minced
- ½ Teaspoon Red Pepper Flakes
- 2 Cups Chicken Broth
- 2 Cups Heavy Whipping Cream

Directions:

1. Start by getting out a large pot to sauté your pancetta, onion and Italian sausage in using medium heat. This should take about five minutes to cook all the way through.
2. Stir your chicken broth, garlic, red pepper flakes, heavy cream, black pepper and Italian seasoning in, and then bring it to a boil.

3. Once it boils, reduce the heat so it simmers for ten minutes. Salt as necessary.

4. Stir in your kale before simmering for another five minutes.

#42 Deconstructed Egg Rolls

Serves: 4

Time: 25 Minutes

Calories: 250

Protein: 33 Grams

Fat: 10 Grams

Net Carbs: 5 Grams

Ingredients:

- 1 lb. Ground Pork
- 1 Egg, Large & Beaten
- 3 Tablespoons Scallions, Chopped
- 1 Tablespoon Sesame Seeds
- 1 Tablespoon Tamari
- 1 Tablespoon Sesame Oil, Toasted
- 1 Tablespoon Chinese Rice Wine
- 1 Teaspoon Ground Ginger
- 4 Cups Cabbage, Shredded
- Black Pepper to Taste

Directions:

1. Get out a skillet and brown your pork using medium heat, and make sure it's cooked all the way through. Don't let it clump up too badly. It should take about five minutes.
2. Add in your egg, and scramble it. This should take another minute.

3. Stir in your tamari, sesame oil, sesame seeds, rice wine, ginger, scallions, and pepper. Reduce the heat so that it simmers for five minutes.

4. Stir in your cabbage, and cook until it's warm all the way through. This should take three minutes.

#43 Chicken Quesadilla

Serves: 4

Time: 50 Minutes

Calories: 619

Protein: 79 Grams

Fat: 35 Grams

Net Carbs: 2 Grams

Ingredients:

- 20 Bacon Strips, Uncured & Center Cut
- 2 Cups Chicken, Grilled & Sliced
- ¼ Cup Ranch Dressing
- ½ Cup Cheddar Cheese, Shredded

Directions:

1. Start by heating your oven to 400, and then line a baking sheet with parchment paper.
2. Lay five strips of bacon on your sheet, and then weave the next five through it in the opposite direction to create a square. Repeat this with the remaining twenty strips to create four. Bake for thirty minutes, and then trim them so they're the same size. Keep the bacon you trimmed to the side for later.
3. Layer your grilled chicken on two of your bacon squares before drizzling it with ranch dressing. Sprinkle your cheese over it, and then top with the remaining bacons square. Bake until your cheese melts, and then cut in half to serve.

#45 Chicken Pad Thai

Serves: 4

Time: 30 Minutes

Calories: 710

Protein: 90 Grams

Fat: 34 Grams

Net Carbs: 8 Grams

Ingredients:

- 1/8 Teaspoon Ginger
- 1/8 Teaspoon Garlic Powder
- 1 Teaspoon Red Pepper Flakes
- 2 Cloves Garlic, Minced
- Sea Salt & Black Pepper to Taste
- ½ Cup Scallion, Chopped
- 1 Tablespoon Rice Vinegar
- 2 Tablespoons Tamari
- 2 Tablespoons Peanut Oil
- 2 lbs. Chicken Tenders
- 3 Eggs, Lightly Beaten
- 1/3 Cup Chicken Broth
- 3 Tablespoons Peanut Butter
- 1/3 Cup Chicken Broth
- ½ Cup Bean Sprouts
- ½ Cup Peanuts, Crushed for Garnish
- 4 Zucchini, Spiralized
- 1 Lime, Sliced into Wedges for Garnish

Directions:

1. Mix your ginger, garlic powder salt and pepper in a bowl, and then toss your chicken tenders in to coat.
2. Heat a skillet over medium-high heat, adding in your peanut oil. Once it's hot, add your chicken tenders in. turn once, cooking all the way through. This should take three minutes.
3. Slice it into ¼ inch slices before setting it to the side.
4. Scramble your eggs in the skillet, cooking for about a minute, and then set them to the side.
5. Turn the heat to medium-low, and then add in your peanut butter, tamari, chicken broth, scallion, garlic, vinegar and red pepper flakes. Stir well, cooking for another three minutes.
6. Add in your chicken, zucchini noodles and scrambled eggs. Mix well before adding in your sprouts, and make sure they're coated in the sauce. Cook for another minute, and serve garnished with lime and crushed peanuts.

Snack Recipes

When you're on the ketogenic diet, it's important that you have snacks to help keep you in ketosis and keep you full. You can meal prep your snacks too!

#46 Pimento Cheese Dip

Serves: 10

Time: 15 Minutes

Calories: 259.2 Grams

Protein: 6.32 Grams

Fat: 24.46 Grams

Net Carbs: 4.03 Grams

Ingredients:

- 8 Ounces Cream Cheese
- 10 Cherry Peppers, Chopped
- 1 ½ Cups Cheddar Cheese, Shredded
- 1 Tablespoon Garlic, Minced
- Black Pepper to Taste

Directions:

1. Heat your garlic in a pan over medium heat, and then add in your cream cheese. Stir to soften, and then mix in your cheddar cheese.
2. Add in your peppers, and then refrigerate until you're ready to serve.

#47 Tuna Deviled Eggs

Serves: 4

Protein: 10.7 Grams

Fat: 11.4 Grams

Protein: 10.7 Grams

Net Carbs: 1.1 Grams

Ingredients:

- 4 Eggs, Hardboiled
- 3 Ounces Tuna, Drained
- 2 Tablespoons mayonnaise
- 1 Spring Onion, Sliced
- 1 Tablespoon Sriracha Sauce

Directions:

1. Peel your hardboiled eggs, slicing them in half. Put your yolks in a bowl. Put your egg whites on a platter.
2. Add the rest of your ingredients to your yolks, and then mash. Make sure it's combined, and then pipe the mixture back into your egg whites.

#48 Liver Bites

Serves: 8

Time: 15 Minutes

Calories: 309

Protein: 27.6 Grams

Fat: 21.1 Grams

Net Carbs: 1 Gram

Ingredients:

- 1 Teaspoon Cayenne
- 2 Teaspoons Paprika
- 2 Tablespoons Swerve
- 24 Chicken Liver Pieces
- 24 Slices Bacon

Directions:

1. Line a baking sheet with foil, and then preheat your oven's broiler.
2. Sprinkle your livers down with seasoning if desired before wrapping them in bacon.
3. Mix your cayenne, paprika and swerve together, seasoning your liver with it.
4. Broil for six to eight minutes.

#49 Cauliflower Fritters

Serves: 6

Time: 15 Minutes

Calories: 99

Protein: 5 Grams

Fat: 7 Grams

Net Carbs: 5 Grams

Ingredients:

- 4 Cups Cauliflower, Riced
- 2/3 Cup Almond Flour
- 1 Tablespoon Nutritional Yeast
- ½ Teaspoon Turmeric
- 2 Tablespoons Butter
- Sea Salt & Black Pepper to Taste

Directions:

1. Mix all of your ingredients except for butter in a bowl, and then mold the mixture into six patties.
2. Melt your butter over medium heat, and then add in your patties. Cook for four minutes each. Make sure to flip them over.

#50 Avocado & Egg Bombs

Serves: 5

Time: 20 Minutes

Calories: 147

Protein: 2.2 Grams

Net Carbs: 1.1 Grams

Ingredients:

- 3 Egg Yolks, Large & Cooked
- ½ Avocado, Large
- ¼ Cup Mayonnaise
- 1 Tablespoon Lemon Juice, Fresh
- 2 Tablespoons Chives, Fresh & Chopped

Directions:

1. Halve your avocados, removing the peel and seeds.
2. Spoon the egg yolk into a bowl, and make sure not to break the whites.
3. Put your avocado and egg yolks in a blender, blending with mayonnaise and lemon juice. Process until smooth, and then pipe it back into your egg whites before serving.

#51 Salmon Mousse Rolls

Serves: 30

Time: 25 Minutes

Calories: 29

Protein: 1.6 Grams

Fat: 2.5 Grams

Net Carbs: 0.7 Grams

Ingredients:

- 1 Tablespoon Dill, Fresh + Some for Garnish
- 8 Ounces Cream Cheese
- 4 Ounces Smoked Salmon
- 2-3 Cucumbers
- ½ Lemon, Juiced

Directions:

1. Slice your cucumbers into thin, long strips.
2. Put your dill, salmon, lemon and cream cheese in a blender, blending until smooth.
3. Spread this mousse over the cucumber, rolling it up tightly.
4. Chill before serving.

#52 Jalapeno Poppers

Serves: 4

Time: 35 Minutes

Calories: 434

Protein: 24.2 Grams

Fat: 35.5 Grams

Net Carbs: 3.5 Grams

Ingredients:

- 12 Jalapeno Peppers, Deseeded
- 1 Cup Ricotta Cheese
- 12 Slices Bacon, Cut Lengthwise
- 2 Tablespoons Cilantro, Fresh & Chopped
- ½ Cup Gruyere Cheese, Grated

Directions:

1. Turn your oven to 400, and then wash your jalapenos. Make sure to pat them dry.
2. Halve and deseed your jalapenos.
3. Mix your cilantro, Gruyere cheese and ricotta together before filling each jalapeno halve.
4. Wrap them with bacon, cooking for twenty to twenty-five minutes.

#53 Caprese Skewers

Serves: 4

Time: 10 Minutes

Calories: 384

Protein: 24.5 Grams

Fat: 27.4 Grams

Net Carbs: 7.1 Grams

Ingredients:

- 4 Cups Cherry Tomatoes
- 4 Tablespoons Basil, Fresh
- 4 Tablespoons Green Pesto
- 4 Cups Baby Mozzarella Cheese Balls
- 1 Cup Olives, Mixed & Pitted

Directions:

1. Mix your pesto and mozzarella together, and then assemble your skewers by alternating your ingredients.
2. Garnish with basil before serving.

#54 Zucchini Fritters

Serves: 6

Time: 15 Minutes

Calories: 96

Protein: 4 Grams

Fat: 7 Grams

Net Carbs: 3 Grams

Ingredients:

- 2 Cups Broccoli Florets, Riced
- 1 Cup Zucchini, Grated & Drained
- 1/3 Cup Scallions, Chopped
- 2 Tablespoons Basil, Fresh & Copped
- 2 Eggs, Beaten
- 1 Tablespoon Nutritional Yeast
- ½ Teaspoon Sea Salt, Fine
- 2 Tablespoons Butter

Directions:

1. Mix all of your ingredients together except for your butter, making sure that it turns crumbly.
2. Mold it into six patties, and then heat your butter over medium heat in a skillet.
3. Once your butter is melted and hot, cook each patty for two minutes per side.

#55 Pizza Fat Bombs

Serves: 6

Time: 10 Minutes

Calories: 28

Protein: 1 Gram

Fat: 3 Grams

Net Carbs: 0 Grams

Ingredients:

- 4 Ounces Cream Cheese
- 14 Slices of Pepperoni
- 8 Black Olives, Pitted
- 2 Tablespoons Sun Dried Tomatoes Pesto
- 2 Tablespoons Basil, Fresh & Chopped
- Sea Salt & Black Pepper to Taste

Directions:

1. Dice up your olives and pepperoni slices, and then add the rest of your ingredients in a bowl.
2. Form into mounds, and garnish with olive, basil and pepperoni to serve.

#56 Guacamole

Serves: 6

Time: 15 Minutes

Calories: 172

Protein: 2 Grams

Fat: 15 Grams

Net Carbs: 11 Grams

Ingredients:

- 4 Tablespoons Lime Juice, Fresh
- 1 Red Onion, Large, Peeled & Diced
- 3 Avocados, Large & Ripe
- Sea Salt & Black Pepper to Taste
- Cayenne Pepper as Needed

Directions:

1. Halve your avocados and then discard the stone. Scoop the flesh from three of your avocado hales, and them ash the flesh.
2. Add in your two tablespoons of lime juice, and dice the rest of your avocado, adding it to another bowl.
3. Add the remaining juices and toss.
4. Combine the mashed avocado with the diced avocado, and chop the onion, adding it in.
5. Season with cayenne pepper, sea salt and black pepper to serve.

#57 Walnut Bites

Serves: 10

Time: 18 Minutes

Calories: 80

Protein: 7 Grams

Fat: 3 Grams

Net Carbs: 7 Grams

Ingredients:

- 2 Tablespoons
- 6 Ounces Parmesan, Grated Fresh
- 1 Tablespoons Butter, Unsalted
- ½ Tablespoon Thyme, Fresh & Chopped

Directions:

1. Start by heating your oven to 350, and then line a baking sheet using parchment paper.
2. Put your butter and parmesan cheese into a food processor blending until smooth.
3. Add in your walnuts and pulse again, and then scoop out the mixture onto a baking sheet. Top with thyme, baking for eight minutes.
4. Allow to cool before storing or serving.

#58 Salmon Bites

Serves: 5

Time: 15 Minutes

Calories: 277

Protein: 19 Grams

Fat: 22 Grams

Net Carbs: 5 Grams

Ingredients:

- 4 Ounces Red Salmon, Cooked & Flakes
- 1 Tablespoons Lemon Juice, Fresh
- 8 Ounces Cream Cheese
- 1 Avocado
- ½ Green Onion, Fresh & Chopped
- 1 Cucumber, Sliced into 10 Pieces (1/3 Inch Rounds)
- Tabasco Sauce

Directions:

1. Start by halving your avocado, and then remove the stone. Scoop the flesh out, placing it in a bowl.
2. Add in your cream cheese before mashing, and then mix in your lemon juice. Season with Tabasco sauce, and then arrange your cucumber slices on a plate. Divide your mixture on top, and then divide your red salmon between them.
3. Garnish with green onions, and store in the fridge.

#59 Smoked Salmon with Dill Spread

Serves: 8

Time: 20 Minutes

Calories: 70

Protein: 5 Grams

Fat: 5 Grams

Net Carbs: 2 Grams

Ingredients:

- 4 Ounces Smoked Salmon
- 4 Ounces Cream Cheese, Full Fat & Room Temperature
- 2 ½ Tablespoon Mayonnaise
- 2 Tablespoons Dill, Fresh & Chopped
- Cucumbers to Serve
- Tomato Wedges to Serve

Directions:

1. Mix your smoked salmon, mayonnaise and cream cheese together in a food processor, pulsing until smooth.
2. Season, and then spread over tomato and cucumber wedges.

#60 Buffalo Chicken Dip

Serves: 4

Time: 30 Minutes

Calories: 286

Protein: 19 Grams

Fat: 20 Grams

Net Carbs: 2 Grams

Ingredients:

- 6 Eggs, Whole
- 6 Ounces Chicken, Cooked
- Water as Needed
- 3 Tablespoons Mayonnaise
- 1 ½ Tablespoon Red Buffalo Wing Sauce, Sugar Free
- 8 Stalks Celery
- ¼ Cup Blue Cheese, Crumbled

Directions:

1. Boil your egg for nine minutes, and then peel the egg. Dice the hardboiled egg, and then cook your chicken. Chop the chicken fine, and then slice your celery into two inch pieces.
2. Take a bowl, adding all ingredients except for your celery. Mix well, and then serve with more hot sauce as needed.

#61 Ranch Dip

Serves: 8

Time: 10 Minutes

Calories: 148

Protein: 0.6 Grams

Fat: 12.3 Grams

Net Carbs: 7.5 Grams

Ingredients:

- 8 Tablespoons Sour Cream
- 2 Tablespoons Ranch Seasoning
- 1 Cup Mayonnaise
- Sea Salt & Black Pepper to Taste

Directions:

1. Mix all of your ingredients into a bowl, mixing until well combined. Cover, and allow it to sit for at least fifteen minutes in the fridge before serving.

#62 Mixed Nuts

Serves: 5

Time: 20 Minutes

Calories: 189

Protein: 6.8 Grams

Fat: 16.5 Grams

Net Carbs: 4 Grams

Ingredients:

- 1 Cup Almonds, Raw
- 1 Cup Peanuts, Raw
- ½ Cup Cashews, Raw
- 1 Tablespoon Butter, Melted
- Sea Salt to Taste

Directions:

1. Heat your oven to 320, and ten grease a baking dish using cooking spray.
2. Put your nuts in your baking dish, baking for ten minutes. Toss your nuts twice, and then add your butter and salt.
3. Return your nuts to the oven, and then bake for another five minutes.

#63 Pepper & Bacon Fat Bombs

Serves: 12

Time: 1 Hour 10 Minutes

Calories: 89

Protein: 3 Grams

Fat: 8 Grams

Net Carbs: 0 Grams

Ingredients:

- 2 Ounces Cream Cheese, Room Temperature
- 2 Ounces Goat Cheese, Room Temperature
- ¼ Cup Butter, Room Temperature
- 8 Bacon Slices, Cooked & Chopped
- Black Pepper to Taste

Directions:

1. Line a baking dish using parchment paper before placing it to the side.
2. Get out a bowl and stir all of your ingredients together.
3. Use a tablespoon to drop small mounds onto your baking sheet, freezing for an hour.
4. Store in an airtight container in the fridge for up to two weeks.

#64 Avocado & Peanut Butter Bombs

Serves: 6

Time: 3 Hours 10 Minutes

Calories: 653

Protein: 12 Grams

Fat: 68 Grams

Net Carbs: 4 Grams

Ingredients:

- ½ Cup Coconut Oil, Melted
- ½ Cup Golden Ghee, Melted
- 1 Tablespoon Vanilla Bean Sweetener, Sugar Free
- 1 Avocado, Peeled, Pitted & Chopped
- 3 Tablespoons Heavy Whipping Cream
- 1 Cup Peanut Butter, Smooth

Directions:

1. Get out twelve mini cupcake tins, lining them with paper cups.
2. Blend your coconut oil, ghee, heavy cream, avocado, peanut butter and sweetener together until smooth.
3. Pour this mixture into the cupcakes, freezing for three hours before serving.

#65 Smoked Salmon Fat Bombs

Serves: 12

Time: 2 Hours 10 Minutes

Calories: 193

Protein: 8 Grams

Fat: 18 Grams

Net Carbs: 0 Grams

Ingredients:

- 2 Ounces Smoked Salmon
- 2 Teaspoons Lemon Juice, Fresh
- ½ Cup Butter, Room Temperature
- ½ Cup Goat Cheese, Room Temperature
- Black Pepper to Taste

Directions:

1. Get out a baking sheet and line it with parchment paper. In a bowl, mix all ingredients together, and then make even mounds on your baking sheet.
2. Refrigerate for two to three hours. Your fat bombs should be firm. They can store in the fridge for up to one week.

#66 Bacon Jerky

Serves: 6

Time: 2 Hours 10 Minutes

Calories: 95

Protein: 9 Grams

Fat: 7 Grams

Net Carbs: 0 Grams

Ingredients:

- 1 Tablespoon Cumin
- 1 Tablespoon Garlic Powder
- 1 Tablespoon Smoked Paprika
- 1 lb. Bacon, Uncured & Center Cut
- 1 ½ Teaspoons Black Pepe
- 1 Tablespoon Chili Powder

Directions:

1. Start by heating your oven to the lowest setting which is usually 150 or 175.
2. Get out a large bowl and mix your cumin, paprika, garlic powder, pepper and chili powder together. Add in your bacon, making sure that they're coated well.
3. Lower your rack to the bottom of your oven, and then put your baking sheets on the bottom rack with your bacon in a single layer.
4. Bake for two hours.

#67 Sour Cream & Onion Pork Rinds

Serves: 6

Time: 2 Hours 50 Minutes

Calories: 278

Protein: 25 Grams

Fat: 19 Grams

Net Carbs: 1.5 Grams

Ingredients:

- 2 lbs. Pork Skin
- 3 Tablespoons Chives, Dried
- 1 Tablespoon Garlic Powder
- 2 Tablespoons Onion Powder
- 3 Tablespoons Sweet Cream Buttermilk Powder
- 1 Tablespoon Garlic Powder

Directions:

1. Start by heating your oven to 350, and then line a baking sheet with parchment paper.
2. Cut your pork skin into one inch squares, and put tem skin side up on your baking sheet.
3. Bake for two and a half hours, and then remove them from the oven. Allow them to cool, and mix your buttermilk powder, onion powder, garlic powder and chives together.
4. Toss your pork rinds in the mixture before serving.

#68 Cheddar Chips

Serves: 4

Time: 10 Minutes

Calories: 457

Protein: 28 Grams

Fat: 38 Grams

Net Carbs: 1 Gram

Ingredients:

- 4 Cups Cheddar Cheese, Shredded
- SEA Salt to Taste

Directions:

1. Start by heating your oven to 350, and then line a baking sheet using parchment paper.
2. Spread your cheese out on the sheet in even mounds.
3. Bake for three to five minutes. You want your cheese to be browned but not burnt.
4. Season with salt.

#69 Whisky Caramelized Onion Dip

Serves: 6

Time: 2 Hours 35 Minutes

Calories: 362

Protein: 4 Grams

Fat: 19 Grams

Net Carbs: 3 Grams

Ingredients:

- 2 Tablespoons Bacon Fat
- ¼ Teaspoon Garlic Powder
- ½ Teaspoon Sea Salt, Fine
- 2 Onions, Cut into ¼ Inch Slices
- 3 Teaspoons Whiskey, Divided
- 1 Cup Sour Cream
- 3 Tablespoons Water, Divided
- ½ Cup Cream Cheese, Room Temperature

Directions:

1. Start by melting your bacon fat using medium-low heat, and then add in your onions once your fat is hot. Cook for three minutes, and break apart your onion pieces as necessary. Stir frequently to keep from sticking. Cook for twenty minutes.
2. Add a teaspoon of whiskey wen your onions get too dry, and alternative between water and whiskey until all of the whiskey is used. Once they're soft, transfer them to a bowl. Put them in the fridge until they're cold.

3. Get out a blender, and blend your cream cheese, sour crema, salt, and garlic powder. Blend until smooth, and then add in your onions. Pulse until it reaches the desired consistency, and then refrigerate for at least an hour before serving.

#70 Parmesan Chips

Serves: 4

Time: 10 Minutes

Calories: 228

Protein: 23 Grams

Fat: 15 Grams

Net Carbs: 2 Grams

Ingredients:

- 10 Ounces Parmesan Cheese, Shredded
- Sea Salt to Taste

Directions:

1. Start by heating your oven to 350, and then line a baking sheet with parchment paper.
2. Put your parmesan in small circles, and then bake for three to five minutes. You want your cheese to brown but not burn, so watch it closely.
3. Sprinkle with salt before serving.

#71 Chicken Ramen Dip

Serves: 4

Time: 1 Hour 5 Minutes

Calories: 156

Protein: 3 Grams

Fat: 16 Grams

Net Carbs: 1 Gram

Ingredients:

- 6 Ounces Sour Cream
- ¼ Cup Cream Cheese, Room Temperature
- 4 Tablespoons Mayonnaise
- 1 Chicken Ramen Seasoning Packet

Ingredients:

1. Mix everything together and then blend with an immersion blender.
2. Refrigerate for at least one hour before serving.

#72 Crab Dip

Serves: 6

Time: 40 Minutes

Calories: 292

Protein: 21 Grams

Fat: 31 Grams

Net Carbs: 2 Grams

Ingredients:

- Grass Fed Butter, Room Temperature
- ½ Cup Red Bell Pepper, Diced
- 1 lb. Lump Crabmeat
- 2 Teaspoons Cajun Seasoning
- 1 Tablespoon Mayonnaise
- 1 Tablespoon Horseradish
- 1 Cup Cream Cheese, Room Temperature
- 1/8 Teaspoon Garlic Salt

Directions:

1. Start by greasing a small baking dish with butter and turn your oven to 350.
2. Mix everything together in a bowl before transferring it to your baking dish.
3. Bake for thirty minutes and serve warm or at room temperature.

Dinner Recipes

Cooking a healthy dinner can be hard with a busy schedule, but with meal prepping, it's easy to stick to your ketogenic diet.

#73 Peanut Sauce Chicken Skewers

Serves: 4

Time: 1 Hour 25 Minutes

Calories: 586

Protein: 75 Grams

Fat: 29 Grams

Net Carbs: 5 Grams

Ingredients:

- 2 lbs. Chicken Breast, Skinless & Chunked
- 6 Tablespoons Soy Sauce, Divided
- 1 Teaspoon Sriracha Sauce + 1/8 Teaspoon
- 6 Tablespoons Toasted Sesame Oil, Divided
- 4 Tablespoons Peanut Butter
- Sea Salt to Taste

Directions:

1. Get out your skewers and allow them to soak for thirty minutes before using them.
2. Turn your grill to low heat, and oil your grill down.
3. Thread the chicken through your skewers, cooking for ten to fifteen minutes. Flip your skewers halfway through the cooking time.

4. While your chicken cooks, mix in your Sriracha sauce, sesame oil, soy
   sauce, and peanut butter. Season with salt, and then serve your
   chicken with the sauce.

#74 Beef Wellington

Serves: 4

Time: 40 Minutes

Calories: 307.5

Protein: 23.6 Grams

Fat: 22.66 Grams

Net Carbs: 2.31 Grams

Ingredients:

- 2 Tenderloin Steaks, Halved
- 4 Tablespoons Liver Pate
- ½ Cup Almond Flour
- 1 Tablespoon Butter
- 1 Cup Mozzarella Cheese, Shredded

Directions:

1. Season your steak with salt and pepper, and add it in your pan. Put it over medium-high heat, and put the butter in a pan, allowing it to melt.
2. Your butter will start to bubble, and then add in your steak. Turn your steak every three minutes to keep it from burning. Each side should be seared, and then put your mozzarella in a microwave safe bowl.
3. Melt it and then stir in your flour, forming a dough with it.
4. Place this dough on parchment paper, and then put another piece of parchment paper on top. Roll it until its flat, and put a tablespoon of pate on the dough. Cut the dough to form a ball around the meat. The pate should be inside, and do this to all slices of your steak.

5. Bake at 400 for twenty to thirty minutes. It should turn golden brown.

#75 Blackberry Spiced Chicken Wings

Serves: 4

Time: 1 Hour 10 Minutes

Calories: 502.7

Protein: 34.5 Grams

Fat: 39.1 Grams

Net Carbs: 1.8 Grams

Ingredients:

- 3 lbs. Chicken Wings
- ½ Cup Blackberry Chipotle Jam
- ½ Cup Water
- Sea Salt & Black Pepper to Taste

Directions:

1. Make your marinade by combining your jam and water.
2. Put your chicken wings in a zipper top bag, and fill it with your marinade. Only fill it two thirds full, seasoning it with salt and pepper. Let it marinate for at least thirty minutes. You can also let it marinate overnight.
3. Turn your oven to 400, and then get out a baking sheet and wire rack.
4. Bake your chicken on the wire rack for fifteen minutes.
5. Brush the marinade over it, baking for another twenty to thirty minutes.

#76 Beef Ragu

Serves: 4

Time: 20 Minutes

Calories: 645

Protein: 37.8 Grams

Fat: 51.1 Grams

Net Carbs: 5.7 Grams

Ingredients:

- 1.8 lbs. Ground Bee
- ¼ Cup Red Pesto
- 4 Tablespoons Parsley, Fresh & Chopped
- 1 Tablespoon Ghee
- Sea Salt & Black Pepper to Taste

Directions:

1. Get out a pan, greasing it with ghee before browning your meat in it. You'll want to cook over medium heat, which will take five to eight minutes.
2. Add your parsley and red pesto in, cooking for five more minutes.
3. Serve warm.

#77 Seafood Casserole

Serves: 4

Time: 40 Minutes

Calories: 391

Protein: 31 Grams

Fat: 28 Grams

Net Carbs: 3 Grams

Ingredients:

- 1 ¼ Cup Heavy Whipping Cream
- 2 Tablespoons Butter, Salted
- ¼ Cup Cheddar Cheese, Shredded
- ½ Cup Swiss Cheese, Shredded
- ¼ Cup Parmesan Cheese, Grated
- 2 Teaspoons Worcestershire Sauce
- ¼ Teaspoon Paprika
- ¼ Teaspoon Nutmeg
- Sea Salt & Black Pepper to Taste
- 1 lb. White Fish, Cut into Pieces
- ½ lb. Large Shrimp, Peeled & Deveined

Directions:

1. Heat your oven to 350, and then get out a nine by thirteen inch baking dish. Spray down with cooking spray, and then get out a microwave safe bowl.
2. In your bowl combine your cream, butter, cheeses, paprika, nutmeg, Worcestershire sauce, sea salt and black pepper. Microwave in thirty

second intervals, stirring in between each one. The cheese should melt, and your mixture should become smooth.

3. Put your seafood in your baking dish, pouring the sauce on top, and then season with salt and pepper again.

#78 Beef Stroganoff

Serves: 4

Time: 25 Minutes

Calories: 369

Protein: 28 Grams

Fat: 25 Grams

Net Carbs: 7 Grams

Ingredients:

- 1 lb. Ground Beef
- 1 Cup Beef Broth
- 1 Tablespoons Butter, Salted
- 2 Cups Mushrooms, Sliced
- 1 Yellow Onion, Diced
- 2 Cloves Garlic, Minced
- 1 Cup Beef Broth
- 1 Cup Sour Cream
- ¼ Teaspoon Xanthan Gum
- Sea Salt & Black Pepper to Taste
- Parsley, Fresh & Chopped
- Grated Parmesan Cheese to Garnish

Directions:

1. Get out a skillet and cook your ground beef over medium-high heat, and stir until it breaks up and is cooked all the way through. This should take seven to ten minutes, and then drain the fat.

2. Melt your butter in the same skillet, adding in your garlic, mushrooms, and onions, stirring frequently so it doesn't burn. Cook until its tender, which should take five to ten minutes.

3. Add in your browned beef, broth, sour cream and xanthan gum, cooking until it thickens and combines. This should take three to five minutes

4. Serve garnished with parmesan and parsley.

#79 Creamy Tilapia Bake

Serves: 4

Time: 25 Minutes

Calories: 369

Protein: 35 Grams

Fat: 25 Grams

Net Carbs: 2 Grams

Ingredients:

- 4 Tilapia Fillets, 4-6 Ounces
- 1 Teaspoon Garlic Powder
- Sea Salt & Black Pepper to Taste
- ¼ Cup Butter, Salted & Room Temperature
- ¼ Cup Heavy Whipping Cream
- ¼ Cup Cream Cheese, Room Temperature
- 2 Tablespoons Lemon Juice, Fresh
- 1 Tablespoon Mustard

Directions:

1. Start by heating your oven to 400 and then get out a nine by thirteen inch baking dish. Put your fillets in a single layer on the bottom, seasoning with salt, pepper and garlic powder.
2. Get out a bowl and combine your butter, cream, cream cheese, lemon juice and mustard. Microwave in thirty second intervals, and stir in between each interval so it doesn't burn mix until smooth. This should take one to two minutes.

3. Pour the sauce in over you fish, cooking for ten to fifteen minutes. It should be cooked all the way through.

#80 Burger Bombs

Serves: 4

Time: 1 Hour 10 Minutes

Calories: 312

Protein: 11 Grams

Fat: 16 Grams

Net Carbs: 18 Grams

Ingredients:

- 12 Slices Bacon
- 12 Cubes Smoked Cheddar Cheese, 1 Inch
- 12 1 Ounce Rounds of Raw Sausage Patties
- Cumin as Needed
- Onion Powder as Needed
- Sea Salt as Needed
- Black Pepper as Needed

Directions:

1. Start by heating your oven to 350, and then put your sausage rounds on a baking sheet lined with parchment paper.
2. Dust them with onion, cumin, pepper and salt.
3. Add your cheese pieces to the middle, forming a ball around each one.
4. Wrap your bacon over each ball, and bake for an hour.

#81 Steak & Broccoli

Serves: 4

Time: 20 Minutes

Calories: 875

Protein: 40 Grams

Fat: 75 Grams

Net Carbs: 10 Grams

Ingredients:

- 1 Yellow Onion
- ¾ lb. Ribeye Steak
- 4 Ounces butter
- 9 Ounces Broccoli
- 1 Tablespoon Coconut Aminos
- 1 Tablespoon Pumpkin Seeds
- Sea Salt & Black Pepper to Taste

Directions:

1. Slice your onions and steak before chopping your broccoli. Chop up the stem as well.
2. Get out a frying pan, placing it over medium heat melt your butter, and then season your meat with salt and pepper.
3. Brown your onion and broccoli in the same pan, adding more butter. Stir in your coconut aminos, transferring the meat back, and then serve with butter and pumpkin seeds.

#82 Butter Scallops

Serves: 4

Time: 20 Minutes

Calories: 306

Protein: 19 Grams

Fat: 24 Grams

Net Carbs: 4 Grams

Ingredients:

- 1 lb. Sea Scallops, Cleaned
- Black Pepper to Taste
- 2 Teaspoons Garlic, Minced
- 1 Lemon, Juiced
- 8 Tablespoons Butter Divided
- 2 Teaspoon Basil, Fresh & Chopped
- 1 Teaspoon Thyme, Fresh & Chopped

Directions:

1. Start by making sure your scallops are dry. Pat them with a paper towel before seasoning them with pepper.
2. Put your skillet over medium heat, adding in two tablespoons of butter.
3. Place your scallops in the pan, and sear each side until they turn a golden brown. It should be about two and a half minutes per side.
4. Set your scallops to the side once they're cooked, and add your remaining six tablespoons of butter into your skillet.
5. Stir in your garlic, cooking for three minutes.

6. Stir in your basil, thyme, and lemon juice before putting your scallops back into the skillet, stirring to coat them.

#83 Fish Curry

Serves: 4

Time: 35 Minutes

Calories: 416

Protein: 26 Grams

Fat: 31 Grams

Net Carbs: 4 Grams

Ingredients:

- ½ Teaspoon Cumin
- 1 Tablespoon Curry Powder
- 1 ½ Tablespoons Ginger, Grated
- 2 Teaspoons Garlic, Minced
- 2 Tablespoons Coconut Oil
- 1 Cup Kale, Shredded
- 2 Cups Coconut Milk
- 16 Ounces Firm White Fish, Chopped into 1 Inch Chunks
- 2 Tablespoons Cilantro, Fresh & Chopped

Directions:

1. Get out a skillet, placing it over medium heat. Melt your coconut oil, and then sauté your garlic and ginger for two minutes. They should be lightly browned. This will take about two minutes.
2. Stir in your cumin and curry powder, sautéing until fragrant. This should take about two minutes, and then stir in your coconut milk. Bring it to a boil, and then turn the heat to low. Allow it to simmer for

five minutes. This will infuse your milk with the spices, and then add in your fish.

3. Cook for about ten minutes. It should be cooked all the way through, and then stir in your cilantro and kale. Allow it to simmer for two minutes.

#84 Buttery Lemon Chicken

Serves: 4

Time: 50 Minutes

Calories: 294

Protein: 12 Grams

Fat: 26 Grams

Net Carbs: 3 Grams

Ingredients:

- 4 Chicken Thighs, Bone In & Skin On
- Sea Salt & Black Pepper to Taste
- 2 Tablespoons Butter, Divided
- 2 Teaspoons Garlic, Minced
- ½ Cup Heavy Whipping Cream
- ½ Cup Herbed Chicken Stock
- ½ Lemon, Juiced

Directions:

1. Start by heating your oven to 400, and then season your chicken thighs using salt and pepper.
2. Put a skillet over medium-high heat and add in a tablespoon of butter.
3. Let your chicken thighs brown until they're gold on both sides. It should take roughly three minutes per side, and then place them on a plate.
4. Add your remaining butter, sautéing your garlic for about two minutes.
5. Whisk in your heavy cream, lemon juice and chicken stock, bringing it to a boil.

6. Once it boils, add I your chicken, and then put your skillet in the oven. Cover it, and braise your chicken for about thirty minutes. It should cook your chicken all the way through.

#85 Bacon & Chicken Burgers

Serves: 6

Time: 35 Minutes

Calories: 374

Protein: 18 Grams

Fat: 33 Grams

Net Carbs: 1 Gram

Ingredients:

- ¼ Teaspoon Sea Salt
- Pinch Black Pepper
- 2 Tablespoons Coconut Oil
- 4 Lettuce Leaves, Large
- 1 Avocado, Peeled, Pitted & Sliced
- 1 lb. Ground Chicken
- 8 Bacon Slices, Chopped
- ¼ Cup Almonds, Ground
- 1 Teaspoon Basil, Fresh & Chopped

Directions:

1. Heat your oven to 350, and get out a baking sheet. Line it with parchment paper, and then get out a bowl.
2. In your bowl, combine your chicken, ground almonds, bacon, basil, salt and pepper, mixing well. Form six patties, and then put a skillet over medium-high heat.
3. Melt your coconut oil, searing your chicken patties until they're browned on each side. This should take about three minutes per side,

and then place them on the baking sheet. Bake them for fifteen minutes so they cook all the way through.

4. Reserve avocado slices and the lettuce leaves for when you're ready to serve.

#86 Easy Paprika Chicken

Serves: 8

Time: 35 Minutes

Calories: 389

Protein: 25 Grams

Fat: 30 Grams

Net Carbs: 4 Grams

Ingredients:

- 4 Teaspoons Smoked Paprika
- 8 Chicken Breasts, 4 Ounces Each & Skin ON
- Sea Salt & Black Pepper to Taste
- 2 Tablespoons Olive Oil
- 1 Cup Sweet Onion, Chopped
- 1 Cup Heavy Whipping Cream
- 1 Cup Sour Cream
- 4 Tablespoons Parsley, Fresh & Chopped

Directions:

1. Start by seasoning your chicken with salt and pepper, and then put a skillet over medium-high heat. Add in your olive oil.
2. Once your oil is hot, sear your chicken until it's cooked almost all the way through, which should take fifteen minutes. Make sure you sear both sides, and then remove the chicken, setting it aside.
3. Add your onion into the skillet, cooking for four minutes. Your onion should become tender.
4. Stir in your paprika and cream, bringing it to a simmer.

5. Add your chicken back into the pan, and then simmer for five more minutes.

6. Stir in your sour cream, and top with parsley before serving.

#87 Easy Dinner Quiche

Serves: 6

Time: 50 Minutes

Calories: 332

Protein: 13 Grams

Fat: 29 Grams

Net Carbs: 2 Grams

Ingredients:

- 1 ½ Cups Colby Jack Cheese, Shredded
- 2 Tablespoons Butter, Salted
- 6 Eggs, Large
- 1 Cup Heavy Whipping Cream
- 8 Ounces Spinach, Frozen & Chopped, Thawed & Squeezed
- Sea Salt & Black Pepper to Taste

Directions:

1. Start by heating your oven to 375, and then get out a cast iron skillet. Grease it with butter before getting out a bowl.
2. Whisk your eggs, cream, cheese, salt and pepper together. Add in your drained spinach, mixing well.
3. Pour this into your skillet, and then bake for a half hour. Your eggs should set.
4. Allow it to stand for ten minutes before serving.

#88 Stuffed Chicken

Serves: 4

Time: 1 Hour 30 Minutes

Calories: 389

Protein: 25 Grams

Fat: 30 Grams

Net Carbs: 3 Grams

Ingredients:

- 1 Tablespoon Butter
- ½ Cup Goat Cheese, Room Temperature
- ¼ Cup Sweet Onion, Chopped
- ¼ Cup Kalamata Olives, Chopped
- ¼ Cup Roasted Red Pepper, Chopped
- 4 Chicken Breasts, Skin On & 5 Ounces Each
- 2 Tablespoons Basil, Fresh & Chopped
- 2 Tablespoons Olive Oil

Directions:

1. Start by heating your oven to 400, and then get out a skillet.
2. Place your skillet over medium heat, melting your butter in it before adding in your onion. Sauté for three minutes. Your onion should become tender.
3. Transfer your onion to a bowl, adding me your cheese, olives, basil and red pepper. Stir until blended, and allow it to sit in the fridge for a half hour.

4. Cut pockets into your chicken horizontally, and stuff them with the filling secure both sides of your chicken breasts with toothpicks so they don't pop open.

5. Get out an ovenproof skillet, putting it over medium-high heat before adding in your oil.

6. Brown your chicken on both sides, which should take five minutes per side.

7. Put your skillet in the oven, roasting for fifteen minutes.

#89 Stuffed Pork Chops

Serves: 4

Time: 50 Minutes

Calories: 481

Protein: 29 Grams

Fat: 38 Grams

Net Carbs: 2 Grams

Ingredients:

- 3 Ounces Goat Cheese
- ¼ Cup Almonds, Toasted & Chopped
- ½ Cup Walnuts, Chopped
- 4 Pork Chops, Center Cut & Butterflied
- 1 Teaspoon Thyme, Fresh &Chopped
- 2 Tablespoons Olive Oil
- Sea Salt & Black Pepper to Taste

Directions:

1. Start by heating your oven to 400, and then get out a bowl.
2. In your bowl make your filling by stirring your almonds, thyme, walnuts, and goat cheese together. Make sure it's mixed well.
3. Season your pork chops with salt and pepper, and stuff them with your filling. Secure the stuffing using toothpicks.
4. Put a skillet over medium-high heat, and then add in your oil. Once your oil is hot, sear your pork chops for five minutes per side.
5. Transfer your pork chops to a baking dish, and then bake for twenty minutes. They should be cooked all the way through.

#90 Chicken Fajita Skillet

Serves: 4

Time: 30 Minutes

Calories: 522

Protein: 35 Grams

Fat: 37 Grams

Net Carbs: 10 Grams

Ingredients:

Fajitas:

- 1 lb. Chicken, Boneless, Skinless & Sliced
- 3 Tablespoons Olive Oil, Divided
- ¼ Cup Cilantro Leaves, Chopped
- 1 Garlic Clove, Minced
- 1 Teaspoon Cumin
- 1 Teaspoon Sea Salt, Fine
- 2 Bell Peppers, Seeded & Sliced Thin
- 1 Yellow Onion, Sliced Thin
- Black Pepper to Taste

Serving:

- 1 Avocado, Sliced
- 1 Cup Cheddar Cheese, Shredded
- 1 Cup Sour Cream

Directions:

1. Get out a large bowl and combine your chicken, olive oil, garlic, cumin, cilantro and salt together. Toss the chicken until it's coated well.
2. Place a skillet over medium heat, and heat up a tablespoon of your oil. Add in your onion and bell pepper, stirring occasionally until they're soft and lightly browned. This should take five to seven minutes, and then transfer the mixture to a plate lined with paper towels so that it drains.
3. Cook your chicken mixture and stir occasionally until the chicken is fully cooked. This should take eight to twelve minutes.
4. Return your bell pepper mixture to the skillet, seasoning with salt and pepper.
5. Serve with avocado, cheese and sour cream.

#91 Pork Loin with a Mustard Sauce

Serves: 8

Time: 1 Hour 20 Minutes

Calories: 368

Protein: 25 Grams

Fat: 29 Grams

Net Carbs: 2 Grams

Ingredients:

- 3 Tablespoons Olive Oil
- 1 ½ Cups Heavy Whipping Cream
- 3 Tablespoons Grainy Mustard
- 1 Boneless Pork Loin Roast, 2 lbs.
- Sea Salt & Black Pepper to Taste

Directions:

1. Start by heating your oven to 375, and then season your pork roast using the salt and pepper.
2. Put a skillet over medium-high heat, adding in your olive oil.
3. Brown your roast on all sides, which should take about six minutes. Put it in a baking dish, and then roast for about one hour. It should reach an internal temperature of 155 at its thickest part. When there is only fifteen minutes left for your roast, put a pan over medium heat, adding in your heavy cream and mustard.
4. Stir your sauce until it simmers, and then reduce your heat to low. Simmer for five minutes. It should become rich and thick, and then

allow your pork to rest for ten minutes before slicing. Serve with your sauce on the side.

#92 Lamb Leg & Sun Dried Tomato Pesto

Serves: 8

Time: 1 Hour 25 Minutes

Calories: 352

Protein: 17 Grams

Fat: 29 Grams

Net Carbs: 3 Grams

Ingredients:

Pesto:

- 1 Cup Sun Dried Tomatoes, Packed in Oil & Drained
- 2 Tablespoons Basil, Fresh & Chopped
- 2 Teaspoons Garlic, Minced
- 2 Tablespoons Olive Oil
- ¼ Cup Pine Nuts

Lamb:

- 2 Tablespoons Olive Oil
- 2 lb. Lamb Leg
- Sea Salt & Black Pepper to Taste

Directions:

1. Put your pine nuts olive oil, garlic, basil and sun dried tomatoes in a food processor, blending until smooth. Set it to the side, and then heat your oven to 400.
2. Season your lamb using salt and pepper, and then get out an ovenproof skillet.

3. Place it over medium-high heat, heating up your olive oil.

4. Sear the lamb until browned on all sides, which will take about six minutes.

5. Spread the pesto over your lamb, and then place it on a baking sheet. Roast until it reaches the desired doneness, which will take an hour for medium.

6. Allow your lamb to rest for at least ten minutes before slicing.

#93 Cheeseburger Casserole

Serves: 6

Time: 50 Minutes

Calories: 410

Protein: 20 Grams

Fat: 33 Grams

Net Carbs: 3 Grams

Ingredients:

- ½ Cup Heavy Whipping Cream
- 1 Teaspoon Basil, Minced & Fresh
- 1 Large Tomato, Chopped
- 1 ½ Cups Cheddar Cheese, Shredded & Divided
- 2 Teaspoons Garlic, Minced
- ½ Cup Sweet Onion, Chopped
- 1 lb. Ground Beef, Lean 75%
- Sea Salt & Black Pepper to Taste

Directions:

1. Heat the oven to 350, and then put a skillet over medium-high heat. Add in your ground beef, browning for six minutes. Spoon the excess fat off, and then stir in your garlic and onions. Cook for four minutes. Your vegetables should become tender.
2. Transfer the mixture into an eight y eight inch casserole dish, and then get out a bowl.
3. Stir together your heavy cream, a cup of cheese, tomato, salt, pepper and basil. Make sure it's mixed well.

4. Pour the cream mixture over your beef mix, and then top with the remaining cheese.

5. Bake for thirty minutes. The cheese should be browned lightly and melted.

#94 Cordon Bleu Casserole

Serves: 8

Time: 45 Minutes

Calories: 587

Protein: 39 Grams

Fat: 47 Grams

Net Carbs: 2 Grams

Ingredients:

- 1 Cup Butter, Salted, Melted + 2 Tablespoons for your Baking Dish
- 4 Cups Chicken Breast, Cooked & Shredded
- 1 Cup Ham, Diced
- 1 Cup Cream Cheese, Room Temperature
- 1 Tablespoon Dijon Mustard
- 2 Tablespoons Lemon Juice, Fresh
- 2 Cups Swiss Cheese, Shredded
- Sea Salt & Black Pepper to Taste

Directions:

1. Start by turning your oven to 350, and then get out a nine by thirteen inch baking dish. Grease it with two tablespoons of butter before layering your ham and chicken in the bottom.
2. Get out a bowl and whisk together your remaining butter, mustard, lemon juice, salt, pepper and cream cheese. Spread this over your ham and chicken, and then sprinkle your Swiss cheese on top.
3. Bake for a half hour. Your cheese should brown, and then allow it to rest for at least five minutes before dishing it out.

#95 Chicken Curry Bake

Serves: 8

Time: 40 Minutes

Calories: 495

Protein: 26 Grams

Fat: 41 Grams

Net Carbs: 5 Grams

Ingredients:

- 1 Cup Mayonnaise
- 1 Cup Sour Cream
- 1 Tablespoon Curry Powder
- 2 Tablespoons Lemon Juice, Fresh
- Sea Salt & Black Pepper to Taste
- 3 Cups Colby Jack Cheese, Shredded & Divided
- ¼ Cup Parmesan Cheese, Shredded
- 3 Cups Chicken, Shredded & Cooked
- 6 Cups Broccoli Florets, Blanched for 2 Minutes & Drained

Directions:

1. Start by heating your oven to 375, and then get out a nine by thirteen baking dish. Spray it down with cooking spray or rub it down with olive oil.
2. Get out a bowl and whisk your sour cream, mayonnaise, lemon juice and curry powder together. Season it with salt and pepper.
3. Add in one and a half cups of your Colby jack cheese with your parmesan cheese, stirring until well combined.

4. Layer your shredded chicken and broccoli on the baking dish, and then top with you sour cream and cheese mixture. Stir together using a fork, and then sprinkle e your remaining cheese on top of the casserole.

5. Bake for thirty to thirty-five minutes. It should be heated up all the way and browned on top.

#96 Coconut Chicken Curry

Serves: 6

Time: 35 Minutes

Calories: 542

Protein: 37 Grams

Fat: 39 Grams

Net Carbs: 11 Grams

Ingredients:

- 2 Tablespoons Coconut Oil
- 2 lbs. Chicken Breasts, Boneless & Skinless Chopped into ½ Inch Chunks
- 1 Yellow Onion, Small 7 Diced
- 1 Red Bell Pepper, Chopped
- 2 Tablespoons Curry Powder
- Sea Salt & Black Pepper to Taste
- 30 Ounces Coconut Milk, Canned & Full Fat
- 1 Lime, Juiced
- 2 Cups Red Cabbage, Sliced Thin

Directions:

1. Get a skillet and place it over medium heat, and then add in your coconut oil to melt it once your coconut oil is melted, add in your cubed chicken, onion, bell pepper, and then season with curry powder. Season with salt and pepper as well, and then cook for five to seven minutes. Your vegetables should soften.

2. Add in your lime juice and coconut mixture before bringing it to a boil for one minute. Reduce the heat to low to simmer, and cover it. Simmer for ten to twelve minutes. Your chicken should be cooked all the way through, and your sauce should thicken.

3. Add in your sliced cabbage, cooking for another three minutes. Your cabbage should soften. Season with salt and pepper again if needed.

#97 Chicken & Green Chili Bake

Serves: 6

Time: 45 Minutes

Calories: 483

Protein: 37 Grams

Fat: 31 Grams

Net Carbs: 3 Grams

Ingredients:

- Butter for Your Baking Dish
- 8 Ounces Cream Cheese, Room Temperature
- 2 Teaspoons Garlic Powder
- 2 Teaspoon Sea Salt, Fine
- 1 Teaspoon Cumin
- 5 Chicken Breasts, Boneless & Skin On (About 3 ½ Ounces Each)
- 4 Ounces Green Chilies, Diced & Canned
- 1 Cup Cheddar Cheese, Shredded

Directions:

1. Start by heating your oven to 375, and get out a nine by thirteen inch baking dish. Prepare your baking dish by rubbing it down with butter.
2. Get out a bowl and mix together your cream cheese, garlic powder, cumin and salt. Add in your green chilies, making sure it's well combined.
3. Lay your chicken breasts in your baking dish, covering with the cream cheese mixture.

4. Top it with your shredded cheese, and then bake for thirty to thirty-five minutes. The chicken should be cooked all the way through, and your cheese should be browned.

#98 Southern Pulled Pork

Serves: 10

Time: 8-12 Hours + 10 Minutes

Calories: 277

Protein: 43 Grams

Fat: 9 Grams

Net Carbs: 2 Grams

Ingredients:

- 3 Drops Liquid Smoke
- ½ Cup Lemon Rosemary Bone Broth (or Chicken Broth)
- ½ Onion, Sliced
- 1 Tablespoon Onion Powder
- 1 Tablespoon Garlic Powder
- 1 Teaspoon Ground Mustard
- 1 Teaspoon Cayenne Pepper
- 1 Tablespoon Paprika
- 1 Tablespoon Chili Powder
- 3 lb. Pork Butt
- Sea Salt to Taste

Directions:

1. Put your slow cooker on low, and then add in your broth, liquid smoke and onion slices. Place your pork butt on top, and then get out a small bowl.
2. In your bowl mix your paprika, chili powder, onion powder salt, ground mustard, garlic powder, and cayenne pepper together. Rub this

mixture over your pork butt, and then cover it. Cook until it shred easily which is between eight to twelve hours. Transfer it to a serving dish before shredding it, and then get out a blender.

3. Blend the juice sand onions together, and then mix the sauce over your pulled pork before serving.

#99 Creamy Chicken & Sausage

Serves: 8

Time: 40 Minutes

Calories: 471

Protein: 49 Grams

Fat: 29 Grams

Net Carbs: 2 Grams

Ingredients:

- 2 lb. Chicken Tenders
- 12 Sausage Links
- ½ Cup Chicken Broth
- 2 Tablespoons golden Ghee
- 10 Sun Dried Tomatoes
- 10 Cloves Garlic, Peeled
- 4 Tablespoons Basil Leaves, Chopped & Fresh
- 2 Tablespoons Oregano, Fresh & Chopped
- 2 Tablespoons Thyme Leaves, Fresh
- ½ Teaspoon Red Pepper Flakes
- 1 ½ Cups Mozzarella Cheese, Shredded
- 1 ½ Cups Heavy Whipping Cream
- ½ Cup Parmesan Cheese

Directions:

1. Start by heating your oven to 350, and then put your sausage links and chicken tenders in an oven safe skillet. Scoot it over to one half of the skillet, and in your other half mix your ghee, garlic close, sun dried

tomatoes and broth. Sprinkle the pan with oregano, basil, thyme and red pepper flakes.

2. Back until it's cooked all the way through, which should take twenty-five minutes.

3. Remove your sausage and chicken, cutting them into pieces before setting it to the side.

4. Remove your garlic and sundried tomatoes to chop them too before putting them back in the skillet.

5. Put your skillet over medium heat before stirring in your heavy cream. Bring it all to a simmer, and then add in your parmesan cheese and mozzarella until it's melted and mixed all the way through. Add your chicken and sausage back in, and add a tablespoon of broth if it's too thick. Continue to do this until it reaches the desired consistency.

#100 Baked Sausage & Haddock

Serves: 4

Time: 55 Minutes

Calories: 477

Protein: 56 Grams

Fat: 23 Grams

Net Carbs: 7 Grams

Ingredients:

- 2 Tablespoons Sage, Fresh & Chopped
- 1 Cup Fennel, Sliced Thin
- 10 Cherry Tomatoes, Halved
- 1 Onion, Quartered
- 1 lb. Bulk Sausage
- 2 Teaspoons Garlic Infused Olive Oil
- 2 Tablespoons Lemon Juice, Fresh & Divided
- Sea Salt & Black Pepper to Taste
- 1 Tablespoon Garlic, Minced
- 1 Tablespoon Lemon Zest, Grated
- 4 Haddock Fillets, 7 Ounces Each

Directions:

1. Heat your oven to 400, and then get out an oven safe skillet.
2. Throw your sage and sausage into the skillet, placing it over medium-high heat. The meat should brown, and make sure it's cooked all the way through. Stir often, making sure to break apart any large

clumping. This should take about five minutes. Place it to the side, but keep the fat in the skillet.

3. Put your fennel into your skillet, adding in your onion quarters and tomatoes. Add in your garlic olive oil, and then season with salt and pepper. Drizzle a tablespoon of lemon juice in the skillet, and then put your skillet in the oven for a half hour. Make sure to stir every once in a while to keep it from burning.

4. Get out a bowl, mixing the remaining lemon juice, zest and minced garlic together. Toss your haddocks in this before setting the fillets to the side.

5. Add your sausage to your roasted vegetables, and then put your haddock fillets on top with the onion quarters between them.

6. Bake for ten minutes, and serve warm.

#101 Seafood Chowder

Serves: 6

Time: 1 Hour 10 Minutes

Calories: 348

Protein: 25 Grams

Fat: 26 Grams

Net Carbs: 4 Grams

Ingredients:

- 3 Tablespoons Golden Ghee
- 1 Ounce Salted Pork
- 1 Teaspoons Garlic, Minced
- ½ White Onion, Diced
- 1 ½ Cups Clam Juice
- 1 Cup Lemon Rosemary Bone Broth (or Chicken Broth)
- ½ Teaspoons Celery Salt
- ½ Teaspoons Tarragon
- ¼ Teaspoon Thyme
- 1 Bay Leaf
- 1 lb. Clams, Minced
- 1 lb. Langoustines, Frozen, Precooked & Defrosted Overnight in the Fridge
- 1 Cup Heavy Whipping Cream
- 3 Dashes Worcestershire Sauce
- Sea Salt & Black Pepper to Taste

Directions:

1. Get out a saucepan, and then melt your ghee using medium heat. Add in your salted pork, garlic and onion, cooking for five minutes. Your onion should soften.
2. Pour in your broth, celery salt, clam juice, tarragon, bay leaf and thyme, and then bring it to a simmer. Once it simmers, reduce the heat to medium-low, allowing it to simmer for a half hour.
3. Add your langoustines and clams to the pot, and then increase the heat so that it comes to a boil. Reduce the heat to low, allowing it to simmer for five to ten more minutes.
4. Add in your Worcestershire sauce, salt, pepper and heavy cream. Let it simmer for another ten minutes before stirring in your salt pork to serve.

#102 Bacon Scallops

Serves: 4

Time: 40 Minutes

Calories: 550

Protein: 66 Grams

Fat: 27 Grams

Net Carbs: 7 Grams

Ingredients:

- 1 lb. Bacon, Uncured & Center Cut
- 2 lbs. Sea Scallops, Fresh & Patted Dry
- ¼ Cup White Wine, Dry
- 3 Tablespoons Golden Ghee
- Lemon Wedges to Garnish

Directions:

1. Line a baking sheet with parchment paper, and then heat your oven to 400.
2. Lay your bacon out on a baking sheets, and then bake for fifteen to twenty minutes. They should be crisp, and then let them cool to crumble
3. Put your bacon grease on in a skillet, heating it up over high heat.
4. Brown your scallops in the grease for three to four minutes per side.
5. Add your wine, and then deglaze your pan. Stir in the ghee to make a sauce.

6. Add in your crumbled bacon, and then add your scallops back in. toss
to coat, and heat for one more minute before serving with lemon
wedges. Squeeze your lemon over it before eating.

#103 Tomato & Saffron Shrimp

Serves: 2

Time: 35 Minutes

Calories: 333

Protein: 45 Grams

Fat: 13 Grams

Net Carbs: 9 Grams

Ingredients:

- 1 Fennel Bulb, Cored & Chopped
- 40 Shrimp, Medium & Cooked
- 4 Tablespoons Golden Ghee
- 4 Cloves Garlic, Minced
- 2 Tomato, Chopped
- 1 Cup Chicken Broth
- 2 Tablespoon Lemon Juice, Fresh
- White Pepper to Taste
- Pinch Smoked Paprika
- Cayenne Pepper to Taste

Directions:

1. Place your ghee in a skillet over medium heat. Once it's hot add in your fennel to sauté until soft. This should take three minutes.
2. Add in your garlic, saffron, shrimp and paprika. Cook until it's heated all the way through, which should take another minute. If your skillet begins to dry out, just add more ghee.

3. Add in your broth, lemon juice, cayenne pepper, tomato, and white pepper. Stir well and bring it to a simmer. Simmer until it reduces by half, which should take about twenty minutes. Serve immediately.

#104 Easy Garlic Shrimp

Serves: 4

Time: 20 Minutes

Calories: 308

Protein: 43 Grams

Fat: 14 Grams

Net Carbs: 4 Grams

Ingredients:

- 4 Tablespoons Golden Ghee
- 4 Cloves Garlic, Minced
- 40 Medium Shrimp, Peeled & Deveined
- Pinch Red Pepper Flakes
- Sea Salt & Black Pepper to Taste
- 2 Tablespoons Parmesan Cheese

Directions:

1. Get out a large skillet and put it over medium-high heat to melt your ghee.
2. Once your ghee is hot, add in your garlic and allow it to cook for one minute. The garlic shouldn't brown, and then add in your shrimp. Cook for two more minutes, and then stir in your salt, pepper and red pepper flakes.
3. Sauté your shrimp until they're cooked all the way through which should take five minutes.
4. Stir your parmesan in before serving.

#105 Avocado & Shrimp Tacos

Serves: 4

Time: 50 Minutes

Calories: 958

Protein: 54 Grams

Fat: 80 Grams

Net Carbs: 4 Grams

Ingredients:

Shrimp:

- 4 Tablespoons Olive Oil
- 2 Teaspoons Lime Juice, Fresh
- 2 Cloves Garlic
- 1 Cup Cilantro, Fresh & Chopped
- ½ Teaspoon Red Pepper Flakes
- 1 Jalapeno Pepper, Halved & Seeded
- 2 Teaspoons Sea Salt, Fine
- 2 Teaspoons black Pepper
- 20 Medium Shrimp, Peeled & Deveined

Taco Shells:

- 2 Cups Cheddar Cheese, Shredded
- 1 Cup Monterey Jack Cheese
- 1 Cup Colby Cheese

For Garnish:

- 2 Avocados, Peeled, Pitted & Chopped

- 2 Tablespoons Red Onion, Minced
- 2 Teaspoons Lime Zest, Grated

Directions:

1. Blend your lime juice, cilantro, garlic, olive oil, salt, red pepper flakes, jalapeno and black pepper together in a food processor.
2. Place this mixture into a zipper top bag, adding in your shrimp, and toss to coat. Allow it to sit for thirty minutes.
3. Preheat your oven and line a baking sheet with parchment paper. Get out a bowl, and combine all of your cheeses, and then form twelve four inch circles on the baking sheet with the mixture. Bake for about five minutes. The edges should be browned.
4. Use a spatula to flip up the form the taco shells.
5. In a skillet, cook your shrimp over medium-high heat for about five minutes. They should be cooked all the way through.
6. Assemble your tacos with all ingredients.

#106 Herb Sirloin Roast

Serves: 6

Time: 1 Hour 10 Minutes

Calories: 590

Protein: 47 Grams

Fat: 43 Grams

Net Carbs: 3 Grams

Ingredients:

- ¼ Cup Olive Oil
- 2 Tablespoons Italian Dressing
- 2 Tablespoons Garlic, Minced
- ¼ Cup Thyme, Fresh & Chopped
- 2 Tablespoons Rosemary Leaves, Fresh & Chopped
- ¼ Cup Basil, Fresh & Chopped
- 1 Tablespoon Sea Salt, Fine
- 1 Teaspoon Black Pepper
- 3 lb. Sirloin Roast

Directions:

1. Get out a container that has a lid, and combine your olive oil, Italian dressing, basil, thyme, rosemary, garlic, salt and pepper together. Place your roast in the mixture, and then make sure it's coated on both sides.
2. Marinate it overnight or at least for an hour.
3. Turn your oven to 350, and then put your meat in a roasting pan. Bake for an hour, and let it stand for ten minutes before slicing.

#107 Citrus & Sriracha Beef

Serves: 4

Time: 20 Minutes

Calories: 503

Protein: 65 Grams

Fat: 23 Grams

Net Carbs: 4 Grams

Ingredients:

- 1 Tablespoon Toasted Sesame Oil
- 2 lbs. Flank Steak, Sliced into Thin Strips
- 1 Red Bell Pepper, Seeded & Sliced into Thin Strips
- 1 Tablespoon Garlic, Minced
- 1 Mandarin Orange, Small & Juiced
- 3 Tablespoons Tamari
- 2 Tablespoon Sriracha
- 1 Teaspoon Sesame Seeds
- 1 Teaspoon Rice Vinegar

Directions:

1. Get out a skillet, and heat up your sesame oil using medium heat. Once it's hot, add in your red bell pepper, garlic, and steak. Cook until the steak is cooked through and your peppers are tender but crisp. This will take roughly three minutes.
2. Add in your tamari, Sriracha, rice vinegar and orange juice.
3. Reduce your heat to low so it can simmer for three to five minutes.
4. Serve tossed with sesame seeds.

#108 24 Hour Spicy Stew

Serves: 8

Time: 24 Hours 10 Minutes

Calories: 208

Protein: 11 Grams

Fat: 16 Grams

Net Carbs: 2 Grams

Ingredients:

- 3 lb. Pot Roast
- 3 Cups Beef Broth
- 1 Tablespoon Tangy Ranch Rub
- 10 Ounce Can of Rotel
- 1 Tablespoon Golden Ghee
- 2 Teaspoons Hot Sauce
- 28 Ounces Diced Tomatoes, Canned & Undrained
- ½ Teaspoon Red pepper Flakes
- 1 Teaspoon Garlic, Minced
- ½ Onion, Chopped

Directions:

1. Turn your slow cooker to low, and then get out your beef. Rub it down with your ranch rub before placing it in your slow cooker. Cove, and cook it for twelve hours.
2. In the morning, shred the meat, and remove excess fat.
3. Add your ghee, hot sauce, broth, tomatoes, rotel, onion, garlic, and red pepper flakes. Cook on low for another twelve hours. Serve warm.

#109 Steak & Cheese Peppers

Serves: 4

Time: 45 Minutes

Calories: 433

Protein: 42 Grams

Fat: 25 Grams

Net Carbs: 6 Grams

Ingredients:

- 4 Green Bell Peppers, Tops Chopped off & Reserved, Seeded
- 1 Tablespoon Golden Ghee
- 1 Tablespoon Garlic, Minced
- ¼ Cup Onion, Chopped
- 1 Tablespoon Olive Oil
- 1 lb. Shaved Steak
- 1 Tablespoon Dijon Mustard
- 2 Tablespoons Mayonnaise
- 6 Slices American Cheese, Divided

Directions:

1. Start by heating your oven to 400, and then get out a baking sheet. Line it with parchment paper, and then place your bell peppers with the cut side up on this sheet.
2. Chop the bell pepper tops, and then melt your ghee over medium-low heat in a large skillet. Sauté your garlic, bell pepper tops and onions until soft, which should take about two minutes.

3. Add your olive oil, and once it's hot add in your steak. Your meat should brown all the way through, which will take roughly two minutes.

4. Reduce the heat to low, and then stir in your mustard and mayonnaise.

5. Add two slices of your American cheese on top of the steak, letting it melt for a minute more. Stir to make sure it's mixed all the way through.

6. Spoon this mixture into your green peppers, and top each pepper with another cheese slice.

7. Bake for a half hour, and serve warm.

#110 Curried Beef

Serves: 4

Time: 40 Minutes

Calories: 432

Protein: 38.75 Grams

Fat: 27.5 Grams

Net Carbs: 3.75 Grams

Ingredients:

- 3 Teaspoons Garlic, Minced
- 1 Tablespoon Coconut Oil
- 1 ½ lbs. Stew Beef Meat
- ½ White Onion, Diced
- 2 Teaspoons Curry Powder
- 1 Teaspoon Cumin
- 1 Teaspoon Sea Salt, Fine
- ½ Teaspoon Chili Powder
- 1 Can Coconut Milk, Refrigerated
- ½ Cup Water
- 4 Ounces Cauliflower

Directions:

1. put you can of coconut milk in the freeze so it's ready to use when you need it
2. Get out a pan, heating it over medium-high heat, and add in a half a tablespoon of coconut oil.

3. Once it's hot, add in your stew meat pieces, and brown it on all sides. It doesn't have to be cooked all the way through at this point.

4. Remove your meat and set it to the side in a bowl, and add another half a tablespoon of coconut oil to your pan, heating it over medium heat.

5. Add in your onion, and then cook for one to two more minutes. The spices should become fragrant, and then add your stew meat back in.

6. Remove your coconut milk from the freezer. Make sure it was in there for at least ten minutes, and then open the can. It should have hardened, so you can easily separate the coconut water at the bottom. Add in the hardened coconut milk to your beef mixture, melting it down.

7. Add your water, and stir until it's thoroughly combined. Cover the pan, and simmer for twenty minutes.

8. Add in your cauliflower, and then cook of ten minutes before covering again. Cook until the sauce thickens into a curry consistency.

#111 Chicken Saag

Serves: 4

Time: 35 Minute

Calories: 307.25

Protein: 24.75 Grams

Fat: 20.25 Grams

Net Carbs: 4 Grams

Ingredients:

- 1 lb. Chicken Thighs, Boneless & Skinless
- 4 Cups Spinach, Frozen
- 2 Tablespoons Coconut Oil
- 1 Roma Tomato, Diced
- 1/3 White Onion, Sliced
- 2 Teaspoons Garlic, Minced
- ½ Inch Piece Ginger, Fresh & Grated
- 2 ½ Teaspoons Cumin
- 2 Teaspoons Turmeric Powder
- ¾ Teaspoon Allspice
- 1 Teaspoon Chili Powder
- 1 Teaspoon Pink Salt
- ¼ Cup Heavy Whipping Cream
- ¼ Cup Sour Cream

Directions:

1. Start by dicing your thighs into bite sized pieces, and then put it to the size. Dice your tomato, and then slice your onions. Thaw your spinach, and then drain it. Set it aside.

2. Heat up a skillet over medium-high heat, adding in a tablespoon of ghee. Add in your skillet, cooking until it's completely cooked through. Set it to the side, and then add another tablespoon of ghee into your skillet.

3. Reduce the heat to medium-low, and then add in your tomatoes and diced onion, cooking for another three to five minutes. The onions should be tender, and your tomatoes should be soggy. Add in your ginger and garlic, cooking for another minute. It should become fragrant, and then add in the chili powder, allspice, salt, turmeric and cumin, cooking for another two minutes.

4. Turn the heat back up to medium, adding your chicken and spinach back in. combine, cooking for two to three more minutes. Your water should have mostly evaporated.

5. Add your sour cream and heavy whipping cream, combining until smooth. Cook for another three to five minutes with a lid before serving.

#112 Easy Spicy Shrimp

Serves: 4

Time: 20 Minutes

Calories: 395

Protein: 48 Grams

Fat: 19 Grams

Net Carbs: 5 Grams

Ingredients:

- 2 Tablespoons Garlic, Minced
- Sea Salt & Black Pepper to Taste
- 2 Teaspoons Turmeric
- Pinch Saffron
- 3 Tablespoons Golden Ghee
- 1 Onion, Chopped
- 4 Tablespoons Sriracha
- 2 lbs. Medium Shrimp, Peeled & Deveined

Directions:

1. Get out a bowl and mix your salt, pepper, saffron, turmeric and garlic together.
2. Get out a skillet and melt your ghee using medium heat before adding in your onion. Cook for three to five minutes. Your onion should soften, and then add in your spices. Cook for another two minutes before adding in your Sriracha.
3. Add in your shrimp, cooking for five more minutes before serving.

#113 Blue Cheese Beef Roll Ups

Serves: 4

Time: 55 Minutes

Calories: 527

Protein: 66 Grams

Fat: 27 Grams

Net Carbs: 1 Grams

Ingredients:

- 1 Tablespoon Olive Oil
- 2 Teaspoon Garlic, Minced
- 2 lbs. Steak, Pounded Thin into 4x4 Inch Pieces
- 1/8 Teaspoon Cinnamon
- 1 Teaspoon Sea Salt, Fine
- 1 Teaspoon Black Pepper
- 2 Teaspoon Rosemary Leaves, Fresh & Chopped
- 2 Teaspoon Thyme Leaves, Fresh & Chopped
- ½ Cup Blue Cheese, Crumbled

Directions:

1. Start by heating your oven to 375, and then line a baking sheet using parchment paper. Soak your toothpicks in water. You'll need ten to twenty of them.
2. Combine your garlic, thyme olive oil, rosemary, sea salt, pepper and cinnamon in a zipper top bag, and then marinate your steak in the mixture for a half hour.

3. Put your steak pieces on a baking sheet, and then put blue cheese in the middle. Roll the up, and use a toothpick to secure it.
4. Bake until it reaches the desired level of doneness, which can be anywhere from ten to twenty minutes.

#114 Cheese Stuffed Meatballs

Serves: 5

Time: 40 Minutes

Calories: 521

Protein: 72 Grams

Fat: 23 Grams

Net Carbs: 4 Grams

Ingredients:

- 1 lb. Ground Beef
- 1 lb. Ground Pork
- 1 Egg, Lightly Beaten
- 1 Tablespoon Water
- ½ Cup Parmesan Cheese, Grated
- ½ Cup Mozzarella Cheese, Shredded
- 1 Tablespoon Garlic, Minced
- 1 Tablespoon Italian Seasoning
- 1 Teaspoon Cajun Seasoning
- 1 Teaspoon Sea Salt, Fine
- 1 Teaspoon Black Pepper to Taste
- 8 Ounces Mozzarella Cheese Ball

Directions:

1. Start by heating your oven to 400, and then get out a baking sheet.
2. Line it with parchment paper, and then get out a large bowl.

3. Combine your mozzarella, egg, pork, beef, water, parmesan, Italian seasoning, Cajun seasoning, salt, pepper and garlic. Mix well, and then form meatballs.

4. Cut your fresh mozzarella ball into cubes to stuff into each meatball before resealing them.

5. Place them on a baking sheet, and bake for twenty minutes before serving.

#115 Philly Meatloaf

Serves: 4

Time: 55 Minutes

Calories: 656

Protein: 56 Grams

Fat: 44 Grams

Net Carbs: 9 Grams

Ingredients:

- 1 lb. Ground Beef
- ½ Yellow Onion, Chopped
- 1 Green Bell Pepper, Seeded & Chopped
- 4 Cups American Cheese, Shredded & Divided
- ½ Teaspoon Onion Powder
- ½ Teaspoon Garlic Powder
- ½ Teaspoon Black Pepper
- 1 Teaspoon Sea Salt
- 2 Tablespoons Worcestershire Sauce
- 1/3 Cup Heavy Whipping Cream

Directions:

1. Start by turning your oven to 350.
2. Mix your Worcestershire sauce salt, pepper, garlic powder onion powder, green bell pepper, beef, onion and heavy cream together in a large bowl.
3. Spread your meatloaf mixture into the bottom of a baking dish, and then top it using two cups of your American cheese.

4. Layer the rest of the meatloaf on top, and then top with the remaining two cups of cheese.

5. Bake for forty-five minutes, and let it rest five minutes before slicing.

#116 Vegetable Fried Beef

Serves: 4

Time: 20 Minutes

Calories: 297

Protein: 42 Grams

Fat: 13 Gams

Net Carbs: 3 Grams

Ingredients:

- 3 Eggs, Large
- 1 lb. Ground Beef
- 1 Tablespoon Tamari
- 1 Tablespoon Peanut Butter
- 1 Cup Pea Pods, Trimmed
- 1/8 Teaspoon Ginger
- 1 Scallion, Sliced
- ¼ Cup Broccoli, Chopped

Directions:

1. In a skillet brown your beef using medium-high heat. It should take about three minutes, and then put it to the side. Leave some of the grease in the skillet, but don't use all of it.
2. Reduce the heat to medium before adding in your eggs, and cook for a minute. Make sure you scramble them.
3. Add your meat back into the skillet, and then add your tamari sauce before stirring well.

4. Add in your pea pods, broccoli, ginger, scallion, and peanut butter. Cover, cooking for five minutes.
5. Stir once more before serving.

#117 Onion & Bacon Meatballs

Serves: 6

Time: 50 Minutes

Calories: 510

Protein: 65 Grams

Fat: 23 Grams

Net Carbs: 9 Grams

Ingredients:

- 1 lb. Ground Pork
- 1 lb. Ground Beef
- 2 Eggs, Lightly Beaten
- 1 Cup Parmesan Cheese, Grated
- 1 Cup Mozzarella Cheese, Shredded
- ¾ Cup Garlic, Minced
- 2 Teaspoon Italian Seasoning
- 2-3 Onions
- 1 lb. Bacon, Uncured & Center Cut

Directions:

1. Start by heating your oven to 350, and then get out a baking sheet. Line it with parchment paper before getting out a large bowl.
2. In the bowl combine your pork, eggs, parmesan, mozzarella, beef, garlic, pepper and Italian seasoning. Make sure all ingredients are mixed well, and then make meatballs that are big enough to fill the onion shells in the next step.

3. Cut the top and bottom off of each onion before separating them into layers. Stuff each onion shell with the meatball, and then wrap it with bacon.

4. Place them on your baking sheet, and bake for a half hour. Serve warm.

#118 Mexican Casserole

Serves: 6

Time: 30 Minutes

Calories: 720

Protein: 60 Grams

Fat: 52 Grams

Net Carbs: 3 Grams

Ingredients:

- 1 Tablespoon Lime Juice, Fresh
- 2 Avocados, Ripened, Pitted, Peeled & Chunked
- ¼ Cup Cilantro, Fresh & Chopped
- ¼ Cup Onion, Diced
- 1 Teaspoon Garlic, Minced
- 1 Tomato, Seeded & Chopped
- ½ Teaspoon Sea Salt, Fine
- ¼ Cup Water
- 2 lbs. Ground Beef
- ¼ Cup Taco Seasoning
- 2 Cups Lettuce, Shredded
- 2 Cups Sour Cream
- 2 Cups Cheddar Cheese, Shredded
- Cayenne Pepper Sauce

Directions:

1. Mash your avocado, lime juice, cilantro, onion, tomato, garlic and salt together to make your guacamole before covering the bowl in plastic wrap. Place it in the fridge as you continue.
2. Get out a medium skillet, and then cook your ground beef using medium heat. It should be crumbled and browned, which will take about ten minutes. Stir in your water and seasoning before reducing it to a simmer. This should take another ten minutes.
3. Get out a nine by nine inch baking dish, putting your meat on the bottom.
4. Top with sour cream and then guacamole.
5. Sprinkle lettuce and cheddar cheese on top before drizzling with cayenne pepper to serve.

#119 Cowboy Ribeye

Serves: 4

Time: 1 Hour 5 Minutes

Calories: 426

Protein: 50 Grams

Fat: 24 Grams

Net Carbs: 2 Grams

Ingredients:

- 1 Tablespoon Sea Salt + A Pinch
- 1 Teaspoon Garlic Powder
- ½ Teaspoon Black Pepper
- 2 lb. Cowboy Ribeye Steak
- 6 Rosemary Sprigs, Fresh & Divided
- 7 Cloves Garlic, Peeled & Divided
- 1 Tablespoon Olive Oil + Additional for Drizzle
- 3 Tablespoon Butter, Room Temperature

Directions:

1. Start by turning your oven to 400.
2. In a bowl mix your garlic powder, salt and pepper before rubbing it over the steak. Allow the meat to rest for thirty minutes.
3. Get out a cast iron skillet and put in five close of garlic and five rosemary sprigs, and then drizzle the olive oil over them, making sure some of the oil gets on the bottom of your skillet as well. Place your meat in the skillet, and put it in the oven to just before your desired doneness. It'll take roughly fifteen minutes to reach medium remove it

from the oven, and then in a different skillet warm a tablespoon of olive oil using high heat.

4. Transfer your steak to this skillet, searing both sides for thirty seconds each.

5. Allow your steak to rest for ten minutes, and get out a small bowl. Mix your butter, remaining rosemary sprig, salt, and two garlic cloves by mashing it together to create a pesto.

6. Spread your pesto over your steak before serving.

Side Dish Recipes

Side dishes don't have to be cooked the day of either. In the previous chapter, you learned how to cook a lot of main dishes, but here are some sides that can be prepared in advance too.

#120 Spiced Beans

Serves: 4

Time: 15 Minutes

Calories: 93

Protein: 2 Grams

Fat: 8 Grams

Net Carbs: 4 Grams

Ingredients:

- 2 Cloves Garlic, Minced
- Red Pepper Flakes to Taste
- Pinch Sea Salt
- 4Cups Green Beans, Trimmed
- 2 Tablespoons Golden Ghee

Directions:

1. Fill a pot with water before bringing it to a boil. Add in some sea salt, and blanch your green beans for three minutes.
2. Plunge them into a bowl of ice water to stop the cooking, and then drain them once cool. Set your green beans to the side.

3. Get out a skillet to melt your ghee over medium heat, adding in your red pepper once hot. Add in your sea salt and garlic too, cooking until it's fragrant. Cook for a minute.

4. Add your green beans in, cooking for another three minutes.

#121 Crab Cakes

Serves: 4

Time: 20 Minutes

Calories: 498

Protein: 38 Grams

Fat: 19 Grams

Net Carbs: 5 Grams

Ingredients:

- 1 Egg, Large
- 1 Teaspoon Mustard
- 1 Tablespoon Lemon Juice, Fresh
- 1 lb. Lump Crabmeat
- 3 Tablespoons mayonnaise
- 3 Tablespoons Coconut Flour
- ¼ Cup Coconut Oil
- Sea Salt & Black Pepper to Taste

Directions:

1. Whisk your egg, lemon juice, mayonnaise and mustard in a bowl.
2. Fold in your crabmeat, and try not to break it up. Add in your coconut flour, and season with salt and pepper. Stir to combine.
3. Form into six patties, and then eat up a large skillet using medium heat. Melt your coconut oil, and cook for three to five minutes per side.

#122 Cauliflower Mac & Cheese

Serves: 4

Time: 40 Minutes

Calories: 315

Protein: 16.5 Grams

Fat: 25.5 Grams

Net Carbs: 5.5 Grams

Ingredients:

Base:

- ½ Onion, Diced
- 2 Slices Bacon, Thick Cut
- 6-8 Cups Cauliflower
- 2 Cloves Garlic, Chopped Fine

Cheese Sauce:

- ¼ Cup Heavy Whipping Cream
- 1 Cup Cheddar Cheese, Shredded
- 2 Tablespoons Butter
- Sea Salt & Black Pepper to Taste

Topping:

- 1/2 Cup Cheddar Cheese, Shredded
- ½ Ounce Pork Rinds, Crushed

Directions:

1. Start by heating your skillet over medium heat, and then heat your oven to 425.

2. Dice your bacon, and separate your cauliflower into macaroni sized pieces. You can do this using a knife or by hand. Add in your bacon, and cook the mixture in the skillet for five minutes. Your bacons should be almost fully cooked.

3. Dice your onion and chop your garlic, adding them to the skillet and cooking for another ten minutes. Your onions should be translucent and your cauliflower should be cooked all the way through. Make sur the cauliflower is al dente so it doesn't over cook when you bake the topping.

4. To make your cheese sauce, combine a cup of cheddar cheese, heavy cream and butter in a saucepan, and then cook over low heat until it's melted and well combined. Season with salt and pepper.

5. Put your cauliflower mixture into an eight by eight inch baking dish, and then pour the sauce over it. Top with your remaining cheddar cheese and pork finds, baking for ten minutes.

6. You'll want to broil for three to five minutes more. The topping should be golden and crisp.

#123 Cauliflower Fried Rice

Serves: 4

Time: 30 Minutes

Calories: 153

Protein: 7.3 Grams

Fat: 9.25 Grams

Net Carbs: 7.75 Grams

Ingredients:

- 1 Tablespoon Garlic, Mined
- ½ Cup White Onion
- 1 Tablespoon Liquid Aminos
- 1 Head Cauliflower
- ½ Cup Frozen Peas & Carrots
- 1 Tablespoon Ghee
- 2 Eggs, Large
- 1 Tablespoon Sesame Seeds
- 2 Teaspoons Sesame Oil
- Sea Salt & Black Pepper to Taste

Directions:

1. Start by putting your cauliflower in small pieces into a food processor, pulsing until it's riced.
2. Heat a skillet over medium-high heat, adding in your ghee.
3. Put your rice into a pan, flattening it out and let it cook for ten minutes.

4. Stir your rice, and then add in your peas, carrots, garlic and onion, seasoning with salt and pepper.

5. Continue to cook for five more minutes, and then push your rice to one side of the pan, and crack in your two eggs.

6. Combine the egg and rice until it's cooked all the way through.

7. Add the sesame oil and soy sauce, mixing until well combined.

8. Garnish with sesame seeds before serving.

#124 Jalapeno & Cheddar Biscuit

Serves: 6

Time: 30 Minutes

Calories: 280

Protein: 8.5 Grams

Fat: 26.2 Grams

Net Carbs: 3.3 Grams

Ingredients:

- 1 ½ Cups Almond Flour
- ½ Cup Cheddar Cheese, Shredded
- 1 ½ Teaspoons Baking Powder
- ¼ Cup Heavy Cream
- 3 Tablespoons Butter, Cold & Cubed
- ¼ Cup Jalapeno, Diced
- 3 Teaspoons Parsley, Dried
- 1 Egg
- Sea Salt & Black Pepper to Taste

Directions:

1. Start by heating your oven to 350, and then put your butter in the fridge. This will keep it cold for when you need it.
2. Whisk all of your dry ingredients together, and then mash your butter into your dry ingredients. You should get a sandy consistency before adding in your egg and cream.
3. Fold your cheese in, and then add in your jalapeno and parsley. Do not mix the ingredients. Folding them in will keep the right consistency.

4. Form six balls, and place them on a prepared baking sheet.

5. Cook for seventeen to twenty minutes, and serve warm.

#125 Cauliflower Salad

Serves: 8

Time: 35 Minutes

Calories: 169.25

Protein: 5 Grams

Fat: 14.6 Grams

Net Carbs: 2.5 Grams

Ingredients:

- ½ Tablespoons Yellow Mustard
- 1 Cauliflower Head, Chopped
- 3 Eggs, Hardboiled
- 4 Strips Bacon, Cooked
- 2 Celery Stalks
- ¼ Red Onion, Medium
- 3 Tablespoons Chives
- ½ Cup Mayonnaise
- ½ Tablespoon Apple Cider Vinegar
- Sea Salt & Black Pepper to Taste

Directions:

1. Start by breaking up the cauliflower head into chunks, and then add it to a microwave safe bowl. Cover the bowl using damp paper towels, and microwave on high for three minutes. You'll need to re-dampen the paper towel, microwaving for another three minutes. Your cauliflower should be tender when you test it with a fork.

2. Dice your hardboiled eggs, celery, red onion, chives and bacon. Add it to the cauliflower, tossing until well combined.

3. Combine your mustard, apple cider vinegar, mayonnaise, and season with salt and pepper.

4. Pour this over your cauliflower mixture, and toss before serving.

#126 Ketogenic Stuffing

Serves: 8

Time: 25 Minutes

Calories: 133

Protein: 6.9 Grams

Fat: 9.5 Grams

Net Carbs: 3.8 Grams

Ingredients:

Sausage:

- ½ Teaspoon Paprika
- Red Pepper Flakes to Taste
- ¼ Teaspoon Black Pepper
- ½ Teaspoon Cayenne Pepper
- ½ Teaspoon Sea Salt, Fine
- ½ lb. Ground Pork

Stuffing:

- 2 Tablespoon Butter
- 1 Cauliflower, Large
- ½ Cup Chicken Broth
- 3 Stalks Celery, Chopped
- 2 Teaspoons Garlic, Minced
- ½ Onion, Diced
- 1 Teaspoon Parsley, Fresh & Chopped
- 2 Teaspoons Poultry Seasoning
- Sea Salt & Black Pepper to Taste

Directions:

1. Start by breaking your cauliflower into chunks using a food processor. Do not rice it! Put it in a bowl.
2. Heat a skillet over medium-high heat, and then add in your sausage and spices. Make sure you cook it all the way through, and break it up as necessary. Transfer it to a bowl once it's cooked.
3. Turn the heat down to medium, and then add in your butter. Add in your onion, garlic and celery, sautéing for two to three minutes. Your onion should be tender.
4. Add in your cauliflower, cooking for two more minutes. Make sure to stir continuously. Add in your broth and remaining seasoning, and then cover it. Cook for another five minutes, and then add your sausage back in.
5. Cook for three to five more minutes. Your cauliflower should be tender, and then season with salt and pepper before serving.

#127 Cabbage Coleslaw

Serves: 6

Time: 10 Minutes

Calories: 266

Protein: 0.6 Grams

Fat: 26.4 Grams

Net Carbs: 3.8 Grams

Ingredients:

- 12 Ounces Green & Red Cabbage, Shredded & Mixed
- 4 Ounces Kale, Chopped
- 1 Cup Mayonnaise
- Sea Salt & Black Pepper to Taste

Directions:

1. Mix all ingredients together before serving.

#128 Creamy Cabbage

Serves: 4

Time: 20 Minutes

Calories: 432

Protein: 4.2 Grams

Fat: 42.3 Grams

Net Carbs: 8.2 Grams

Ingredients:

- 2 Ounces Butter
- 8 Tablespoons Parsley, Fresh & Chopped Fine
- 1 ¼ Cups Coconut Cream
- 1 ½ lb. Green Cabbage, Shredded
- Sea Salt & Black Pepper to Taste

Directions:

1. Heat your butter in a skillet, adding in your cabbage and sauté until its golden brown.
2. Stir in your cream, bringing it to a simmer.
3. Add your salt and pepper, and then garnish with parsley before serving.

#129 Green Beans & Roasted Onions

Serves: 6

Time: 25 Minutes

Calories: 214

Protein: 8.3 Grams

Fat: 19.4 Grams

Net Carbs: 3.4 Grams

Ingredients:

- 1 Yellow onions, Sliced into Rings
- ½ Teaspoon Onion Powder
- 2 Tablespoons Coconut flour
- ½ Teaspoon Sea Salt, Fine
- 1 ½ lbs. Green Beans, Fresh, Trimmed & Chopped

Directions:

1. Get out a large bowl and mix your coconut flour with your onion powder, and then add in your onion rings. Make sure they're coated well, and then spread them out on a baking sheet that's been lined with parchment paper. Top with oil, baking at 400 for ten minutes.
2. Parboil the green beans for three to five minutes in boiling water, and serve with your baked onion rings, seasoned with garlic powder if desired.

#130 Red Coleslaw

Serves: 4

Time: 10 Minutes

Calories: 406

Protein: 2.2 Grams

Fat: 40.4 Grams

Net Carbs: 5.2 Grams

Ingredients:

- 1 2/3 lbs. Red Cabbage, Shredded
- 1 ¼ Cup Mayonnaise
- 2 Teaspoons Caraway Seeds, Ground
- 1 Tablespoon Whole Grain Mustard
- Sea Salt & Black Pepper to Taste

Directions:

1. Mix all ingredients together, and let sit for at least ten minutes before serving.

#131 Portobello Mushrooms

Serves; 4

Time: 20 Minutes

Calories: 154

Protein: 6.7 Grams

Fat: 10.4 Grams

Net Carbs: 2.2

Ingredients:

- 12 Cherry Tomatoes
- 2 Ounces Scallions
- 4 Portabella Mushrooms, Stemmed & Removed
- 4 ¼ Ounces Butter
- Sea Salt & Black Pepper to Taste

Directions:

1. Get out a skillet and put your butter in it, placing it over medium heat.
2. Add in your mushrooms, and sauté for three minutes.
3. Stir in your scallions and cherry tomatoes, cooking for another five minutes.
4. Season with salt and pepper as needed.

#132 Easy Fried Cabbage

Serves: 4

Time: 25 Minutes

Calories: 199

Protein: 2.4 Grams

Fat: 17.4 Grams

Net Carbs: 5.4 Grams

Ingredients:

- 1 ½ lbs. Cabbage, shredded
- 3 Ounces Butter
- 1 Dollop Whipped Cream
- Sea Salt & Black Pepper to Taste

Directions:

1. Melt your butter in a skillet, and then add in your cabbage. Cook for fifteen minutes. Your cabbage should be a golden brown.
2. Season with salt and pepper, and serve with cream.

#133 Ranch Broccoli Bites

Serves: 4

Time: 55 Minutes

Calories: 312

Protein: 18 Grams

Fat: 26 Grams

Net Carbs: 4 Grams

Ingredients:

- 8 Ounces Bacon, Uncured & Center Cut
- ¾ Cup Sour Cream
- 1 Cup Cheddar Cheese, Shredded
- 2 Tablespoons Mayonnaise
- 2 Tablespoons Ranch Rub
- 4 Cups Broccoli Florets

Directions:

1. Start by heating your oven to 400, and then line a baking sheet using parchment paper.
2. Put your bacon on the baking sheet, and then bake for fifteen to twenty minutes.
3. Put your bacon to the side before pulling out a bowl. Mix your rub, sour cream and mayonnaise together. Make sure it's mixed well.
4. Place your broccoli in a baking dish, and pour in your sour cream mixture. Make sure to stir well. Top with cheddar cheese, and bake for a half hour.
5. Crumble your bacon over it before serving.

#134 Buttered Green Beans

Serves: 4

Time: 15 Minutes

Calories: 93

Protein: 2 Grams

Fat: 8 Grams

Net Carbs: 4 Grams

Ingredients:

- 2 Tablespoons Golden Ghee
- 4 Cups Green Beans, Trimmed
- 2 Cloves Garlic, Minced
- Pinch Red Pepper Flakes
- Sea Salt to Taste

Directions:

1. Put a pot of water over high heat and salt it. Add in your green beans once it reaches a boil, cooking for three minutes.
2. Make sure you have a bowl of ice water ready, and then drain your green beans before plunging them into your ice water. This will stop the cooking, and then drain them once they're cool. Set them to the side.
3. Take a skillet and place it over medium heat, and then add in your red pepper, salt and garlic. Cook until soft, which will take a full minute.
4. Add in your green beans, cooking for another three minutes.

#135 Creamed Spinach & Peppers

Serves: 8

Time: 20 Minutes

Calories: 237

Protein: 4 Grams

Fat: 23 Grams

Net Carbs: 4 Grams

Ingredients:

- 10 Ounces Baby Spinach, Chopped
- 3 Tablespoons Golden Ghee
- 8 Ounces Artichoke Hearts, Jarred, Drained & Chopped
- ½ Teaspoon Nutmeg
- 8 Ounces Cream Cheese, Room Temperature & Chopped
- ½ Red Bell Pepper, Chopped
- 2 Tablespoons Roasted Garlic
- ¼ Cup Mayonnaise
- ¼ Teaspoon Sea Salt, Fine
- 2 Tablespoons Heavy Whipping Cream
- ¼ Cup Parmesan Cheese, Shredded

Directions:

1. Get out a skillet, and then melt your ghee using medium-high heat.
2. Add your spinach once your skillet is hot, and then add your red bell pepper and artichokes. Sauté until your spinach is fully wilted. This should take five to ten minutes.

3. Turn the heat to low, and then add in your cream cheese. Stir until it's melted into your vegetables, and then add in your nutmeg, salt, mayonnaise and pesto. Stir in your heavy cream as needed to thin the mixture, and cook until completely heated. This should take another minute.

4. Top with parmesan before serving.

#136 Garlic Green Beans

Serves: 8

Time: 20 Minutes

Calories: 104

Protein: 4 Grams

Fat: 9 Grams

Net Carbs: 1 Gram

Ingredients:

- 2 lbs. Green Beans, Stemmed
- 4 Tablespoons Olive Oil
- 2 Teaspoons Garlic, Minced
- ½ Cup Parmesan Cheese, Grated Fresh
- Sea Salt & Black Pepper to Taste

Directions:

1. Start by heating your oven to 425, and then get out a baking sheet. Line it with foil, and then get out a bowl.
2. Toss your olive oil, garlic and green beans together.
3. Season with salt and pepper, and then spread them onto the baking sheet. Roast for ten minutes. Stir once in this time, and then top with parmesan cheese.

#137 Asparagus & Walnuts

Serves: 8

Time: 15 Minutes

Calories: 124

Protein: 3 Grams

Fat: 12 Grams

Net Carbs: 2 Grams

Ingredients:

- 3 Tablespoons Olive Oil
- 1 ½ lbs. Asparagus, Trimmed
- ½ Cup Walnuts, Chopped
- Sea Salt & Black Pepper to Taste

Directions:

1. Put your oil in a skillet, placing it over medium-high heat. Sauté your asparagus until tender and browned lightly. This should take roughly five minutes.
2. Season with salt and pepper, and then remove it from heat.
3. Toss with your walnuts before serving.

#138 Cheesy Brussel Sprouts

Serves: 8

Time: 45 Minutes

Calories: 299

Protein: 12 Grams

Fat: 11 Grams

Net Carbs: 4 Grams

Ingredients:

- ¾ Cup Heavy Whipping Cream
- 1 Cup Swiss Cheese, Shredded & Divided
- 8 Bacon Slices
- 1 lb. Brussel Sprouts, Blanched for 10 Minutes & Quartered

Directions:

1. Heat your oven to 400, and then get out a skillet. Place your skillet over medium-high heat, and then cook your bacon until its crisp. This should take roughly six minutes.
2. Reserve a tablespoon of the fat, using it to grease a casserole dish. Chop your bacon before setting it to the side.
3. Toss your Brussel sprouts with your bacon and a half a cup of cheese, placing this mixture into your casserole dish. Pour in your heavy cream, topping with the remaining cheese.
4. Bake for twenty minutes. Your vegetables should be heated through, and your cheese should be melted and browned lightly.

#139 Cheesy Cauliflower Mash

Serves: 4

Time: 20 Minutes

Calories: 183

Protein: 8 Grams

Fat: 15 Grams

Net Carbs: 4 Grams

Ingredients:

- 1 Head Cauliflower, Roughly Chopped
- ½ Cup Cheddar Cheese, Shredded
- 2 tablespoons Butter, Room Temperature
- ¼ Cup Heavy Whipping Cream
- ½ Cup Cheddar Cheese, Shredded
- Sea Salt & Black Pepper to Taste

Directions:

1. Put out a saucepan over high heat, filling it three quarters the way full with water. Bring it to a boil, and then blanch your cauliflower until its tender. This should take five minutes, and then drain.
2. Transfer it to a food processor, adding in your heavy cream, butter and cheese. Puree until creamy and whipped. Season with salt and pepper.

#140 Parmesan Zucchini

Serves: 4

Time: 25 Minutes

Calories: 94

Protein: 4 Grams

Fat: 8 Grams

Net Carbs: 1 Grams

Ingredients:

- 2 Tablespoons Butter
- ½ Cup Parmesan Cheese, Freshly Grated
- 4 Zucchini, Sliced into ¼ Inch Thick Rounds
- Black Pepper to Taste

Directions:

1. Place a skillet over medium-high heat, melting your butter before adding in your zucchini.
2. Sauté until it's lightly browned and tender, which should take about five minutes.
3. Spread your zucchini out in your skillet, sprinkling your parmesan over it.
4. Cook without stirring until the parmesan melts. It should take about five minutes.

#141 Camembert Mushrooms

Serves: 4

Time: 20 Minutes

Calories: 161

Protein: 9 Grams

Fat: 13 Grams

Net Carbs: 3 Grams

Ingredients:

- 2 Tablespoons Butter
- 4 Ounces Camembert Cheese, Diced
- 1 lb. Mushrooms, Halved
- 2 Teaspoons Garlic, Minced
- Black Pepper to Taste

Directions:

1. Place a skillet over medium heat, and then melt your butter.
2. Add in your garlic, cooking for three minutes.
3. Add in your mushrooms, sautéing until tender. This should take about ten minutes.
4. Add in your cheese, cooking for another two minutes. It should melt.
5. Season with pepper before serving.

Dessert Recipes

Dessert can be hard when you're on a diet, and usually it isn't a temptation you can afford if you want to shed those extra pounds. Luckily, with the ketogenic diet there are various healthy dessert recipes to choose from.

#142 Blackberry & Chia Pudding

Serves: 4

Time: 45 Minutes

Calories: 437

Protein: 8 Grams

Fat: 38 Grams

Net Carbs: 8 Grams

Ingredients:

- ½ Cup Chia Seeds
- 1 Cup Blackberries, Fresh
- 2 Teaspoons Liquid Sweetener
- 2 Cups Coconut Milk, Full Fat & Unsweetened
- 2 Teaspoons Vanilla Extract, pure

Directions:

1. Blend your liquid sweetener, vanilla, and coconut milk into a blender. The mixture should become thick, and then add in your blackberries. Blend until smooth.
2. Refrigerate for at least a half hour to set, and it can keep up to three days in the fridge.

#143 Key Lime Cheesecake Cups

Serves: 12

Time: 40 Minutes

Calories: 279

Protein: 6 Grams

Fat: 27 Grams

Net Carbs: 2 Grams

Ingredients:

Crust:

- 1 Cup Almonds, Raw
- 2 Tablespoons Swerve
- ½ Cup Butter, Salted & Melted

Filling:

- 16 Ounces Cream Cheese, Room Temperature
- 2 Eggs, Large
- ½ Cup Swerve
- 2 Teaspoons Vanilla Extract, Pure
- 2 Limes, Juiced & Zested

Directions:

1. Start by heating your oven to 375. Get out a muffin tin lining it with paper cups.
2. Place your almonds in a blender, blending until finely ground. Add in your sweetener and butter, mixing until it's well combined.
3. Press this mixture into the cups at the bottom, baking for five minutes.

4. Blend your cream cheese, eggs, lime juice, lime zest, vanilla and sweetener together in a blender until well combined.

5. Divide the filling between your crusts, baking for fifteen to twenty minutes more, and then refrigerate for at least an hour before serving. You can also freeze these.

#144 Almond & Caramel Bars

Serves: 12

Time: 40 Minutes

Calories: 229

Protein: 4 Grams

Fat: 21 Grams

Net Carbs: 3 Grams

Ingredients:

- 6 Tablespoons Butter, Salted 7 Melted + More for Your Dish
- 1 Cup Flaked Coconut, Unsweetened
- 1 Cup Almonds, Sliced
- ¾ Cup Almond Flour
- ½ Cup Swerve
- 1 Teaspoon Sea Salt
- 1 Cup Chocolate Chips, Sugar Free
- ½ Teaspoon Baking Soda
- 1 Cup Hot Caramel Sauce (Optional & Keto Friendly Needed)

Directions:

1. Start by heating your oven to 350, and then grease a baking dish using butter.
2. Get out your food processor, combining your almond flour, coconut, almonds, Swerve, salt, baking soda and six tablespoons of melted butter. Pulse until the mixture becomes crumbly, and then fold in your chocolate chips. Press this batter into your baking dish.
3. Bake for fifteen to twenty minutes. It should become golden.

4. Pour your caramel sauce over it, and allow it to rest for ten minutes. Remember that your caramel sauce has to be keto friendly.

#145 Cheesy Raspberry Pops

Serves: 8

Time: 20 Minutes

Calories: 166

Protein: 0.8 Grams

Fat: 17 Grams

Net Carbs: 2 Grams

Ingredients:

- ¼ Cup Cream Cheese
- ¼ Cup Raspberries, Fresh & Chopped
- 4 Tablespoons Heavy Cream
- 4 Tablespoons Coconut Oil
- 4 Tablespoons Butter
- 1 Teaspoon Vanilla Extract, Pure

Directions:

1. Put your coconut oil, butter and cream cheese in a bowl. Microwave for ten second intervals, and stir until it's melted.
2. Add in your heavy cream, and then fold in your raspberries.
3. Stir in your vanilla extract, and then pour into sixteen ice cube trays compartments. Chill for two hours before serving.

#146 Sage & Blackberry Ice Pops

Serves: 8

Time: 5 Hours + Freezing Time

Calories: 10

Protein: 0 Grams

Fat: 0 Grams

Net Carbs: 1 Gram

Ingredients:

- 1 Cup Blackberries
- 2 Sage Leaves, Fresh
- ½ Cup Water
- 1 Teaspoon Vanilla Bean Sweetener, Sugar Free

Directions:

1. Blend all ingredients together before pour into ice pop molds, and then freezing overnight.

#147 Lime & Strawberry Sorbet

Serves: 6

Time: 5 Minutes + Freezing Time

Calories: 104

Protein: 5 Grams

Fat: 8 Grams

Net Carbs: 4 Grams

Ingredients:

- 3 Cups Strawberries, Chopped
- 1 Cup Heavy Whipping Cream
- 1 Lime, Zested
- 3 Tablespoons Gelatin
- 2 Tablespoons Vanilla Bean Sweetener, Sugar Free

Directions:

1. Get out a blender and blend all ingredients together until its thick like whipped cream.
2. Pour this mixture into your ice cream maker, following manufacturer's instructions for sorbet.
3. Freeze for at least two hours before serving.

#148 Chocolate Bacon

Serves: 6

Time: 30 Minutes

Calories: 479

Protein: 30 Grams

Fat: 39 Grams

Net Carbs: 1 Gram

Ingredients:

- 1 lb. Bacon, Center Cut & Uncured
- 2 Tablespoons Golden Ghee
- 1 Ounce Chocolate, Unsweetened
- 1 Tablespoon Heavy Whipping Cream
- 1 Tablespoon Vanilla Bean Sweetener, Sugar Free

Directions:

1. Start by heating your oven to 400, and then get out two baking sheets. Line them with parchment paper, and then put your bacon in a single layer on both sheets. Cook for fifteen to twenty minutes, and drain your bacon using paper towels.
2. Get out a microwave safe bowl, and then combine your chocolate and ghee, microwaving for fifteen second intervals and stirring in between until it's a smooth, soft mixture. This will take three to four intervals. Add in your heavy cream and sweetener, making sure it's mixed well and smooth.

3. Put your bacon on your parchment paper, and then drizzle your chocolate over one third of each slice. Refrigerate your slices for five minutes before serving. Store in the fridge.

#149 Frozen Black Forest Pudding

Serves: 8

Time: 30 Minutes + Freezing Time

Calories: 166

Protein: 4 Grams

Fat: 16 Grams

Net Carbs: 4 Grams

Ingredients:

- 2 Cups Heavy Whipping Cream
- 1 Cups Almond Milk, Unsweetened
- 6 Cherries, Pitted & Chopped
- 1 Cup Cocoa Powder, Unsweetened
- 2 Pinches Sea Salt
- 4 Egg Yolks, Large
- ½ Cup Vanilla Bean Sweetener, Sugar Free

Directions:

1. Start by getting out a medium saucepan, and then place it over medium heat. Heat in your cherries, heavy cream, almond milk, cocoa powder, and salt until hot. This should take about three minutes, and then remove your cherries using a slotted spoon. Set your cherries to the side.
2. Get out a bowl and beat your egg yolks, and pour them into the hot cream while mixing constantly.

3. Pour this mixture back into your pot, cooking while stirring constantly until it's thicken enough to coat the back of your spatula. This should take about fifteen minutes, and then you can add in the sweetener.

4. Pour this mixture into an airtight container, and then refrigerate for two hours.

5. Pour it into your ice cream maker, following manufacturer's instructions.

6. Fold in your chopped cherries once your ice cream is done, and freeze for at least three hours before serving.

#150 Lemon Curd Tarts

Serves: 6

Time: 40 Minutes + Time to Chill

Calories: 296

Protein: 5 Grams

Fat: 30 Grams

Net Carbs: 1 Gram

Ingredients:

- ¾ Cup Almond Meal
- 4 Egg Yolks, Large
- 1 Stick Butter + 3 Tablespoons, Melted & Divided
- 3 Lemons, Zested
- ½ Cup Lemon Juice, Fresh
- ¼ Cup Vanilla Bean Sweetener, Sugar Free

Directions:

1. Get out twelve mini muffin tins, lining them with paper cups.
2. Get out a bowl, and mix three tablespoons of butter with your almond meal, pressing this to a crust in the bottom of your muffin cups.
3. Pull out your blender, blending your lemon zest, lemon juice, yolks, melted butter and sweetener until smooth.
4. Transfer the mixture into a saucepan, cooking over low heat. Stir constantly for fifteen minutes. It should thicken
5. Pour this filling into your muffin cups, making sure to cover the crust fully.
6. Cover with plastic wrap before allowing it to set in the fridge overnight.

#151 Frozen Pumpkin Latte

Serves: 4

Time: 25 Minutes + Freezing Time

Calories: 93

Protein: 2 Grams

Fat: 8 Grams

Net Carbs: 3 Grams

Ingredients:

- ½ Cup Heavy Whipping Cream
- ½ Cup Pumpkin Puree, Pure
- ¼ Teaspoon Nutmeg
- ½ Teaspoon Cinnamon
- 2 Tablespoons Espresso, Cold
- ¼ Teaspoon Ginger
- ¼ Teaspoon Allspice
- 1/8 Teaspoon Cloves
- 2 Egg Yolks, Large
- 3 Tablespoons Vanilla Bean Sweetener, Sugar Free
- 1 Tablespoon Orange Zest

Directions:

1. Start by getting out a medium saucepan, and mix your heavy cream, pumpkin ground spices and espresso together over medium heat for about three minutes. It should be hot all the way through.
2. Get out a small bowl and beat your egg yolks.

3. Take the hot pumpkin mixture and pour them into the egg yolks while whisking constantly. Make sure you do this slowly so that your eggs don't scramble.

4. Pour this mixture back into your pot, cooking while you stir. Scrape the sides, and make sure it's thick enough to coat the back of your spatula. This should take about fifteen minutes, and add in your orange zest and sweetener once it's thick.

5. Pour this mixture into an airtight container, refrigerating for two hours until its cold.

6. Transfer this mixture to the ice cream, and then pour it into the ice cream maker, following your manufacturer's instructions.

#152 Miniature Coconut Pies

Serves: 12

Time: 50 Minutes

Calories: 174

Protein: 3 Grams

Fat: 13 Grams

Net Carbs: 3 Grams

Ingredients:

- 1 Tablespoon Coconut Oil
- 2 Eggs, Large
- 1 Cup Coconut Flour
- ½ Cup Golden Ghee, Melted
- 1 Cup Coconut Cream, Unsweetened
- 3 Tablespoons Vanilla Bean Sweetener, Sugar Free
- ¼ Cup Coconut, Shredded & Unsweetened

Directions:

1. Start by eating your oven to 350, and then get out twelve miniature muffin tins. Coat them with coconut oil.
2. Get out a small bowl and whisk together your eggs, ghee, coconut flour and a tablespoon of sweetener until well combined.
3. Divide this mixture between your muffin cups, patting it into the bottom.
4. Bake for ten minutes, and make sure they have time to cool completely before removing them from the muffin tins. This makes your coconut pie shells.

5. Combine your coconut cream, shredded coconut and two tablespoons of sweetener in another bowl, making sure it's well combined.

6. Top each pie shell with a tablespoon of this mixture, chilling it for a half hour before serving.

#153 Peppermint Fudge Bombs

Serves: 10

Time: 40 Minutes

Calories: 117

Protein: 0 Grams

Fat: 12 Grams

Net Carbs: 1 Gram

Ingredients:

- 1/3 Cup Coconut Oil, Melted
- 3 Tablespoons Vanilla Bean Sweetener, Sugar Free
- 1 Ounce Chocolate, Unsweetened
- 2 Tablespoons Golden Ghee
- 1 Teaspoon Mint Extract
- 2 Tablespoon Heavy Whipping Cream, Divided

Directions:

1. Get out ten mini cupcake tins, and then line them with paper cups.
2. Get out a blender and blend your coconut oil, two tablespoons of sweetener, a tablespoon of heavy cream and your mint extract until thick. This should take about thirty seconds, and then pour the mixture into your muffin cups. Make sure they're filled halfway full. Put them in the freezer.
3. Combine your chocolate and ghee in a microwave safe bowl, and then microwave for fifteen seconds at a time. Stir in between, and continue until it's melted and smooth. Mix in a tablespoon of sweetener and a tablespoon of heavy cream, continuing to mix until it's smooth.

4. Fill your cupcake tins the rest of the way with this mixture, freezing for thirty minutes before serving.

#154 Peanut Butter Fudge Bombs

Serves: 10

Time: 40 Minutes

Calories: 102

Protein: 2 Grams

Fat: 10 Grams

Net Carbs: 1 Gram

Ingredients:

- 4 Tablespoons Golden Ghee
- ¼ Cup Peanut Butter, Smooth
- 1 ½ Tablespoons Vanilla Bean Sweetener, Sugar Free, Divided
- 1 Ounce Chocolate, Unsweetened
- 1 Tablespoon Heavy Whipping Cream

Directions:

1. Get out ten mini cupcake tins, lining them with paper cups.
2. Mix your peanut butter, two tablespoons of ghee, and a half a tablespoon of sweetener until smooth. Microwave it in a bowl for ten seconds at a time, mixing in between until smooth. Pour this mixture into your tins, filling them halfway up. Place them in the freezer for now.
3. In another bowl that's microwave safe, combine the rest of your ghee and chocolate, microwaving it in ten second intervals. Stir after each one until your mixture becomes combined and soft.
4. Mix in your sweetener and remaining cream, mixing until combined and smooth.

5. Remove the tins from the freezer, and then fill them up the rest of the way with this mixture.

6. Freeze for a half hour before serving.

#155 Cookie Dough Bombs

Serves: 12

Time: 1 Hour 10 Minutes

Calories: 167

Protein: 2.3 Grams

Fat: 17 Grams

Net Carbs: 1.2 Grams

Ingredients:

- 8 Ounces Cream Cheese, Room Temperature
- ½ Cup Almond Flour
- ¼ Cup Erythritol
- 8 Tablespoons Butter, Room Temperature
- 25 Drops Liquid Stevia
- ¼ Teaspoon Vanilla Extract, Pure
- ¼ Teaspoon Sea Salt, Fine
- ¼ Cup Keto Chocolate Chips

Directions:

1. Start by combing your cream cheese and butter together using a hand mixer.
2. Add in your stevia, Erythritol, vanilla extract, almond flour and sea salt. Mix well.
3. Fold in your chocolate chips, and then refrigerate for an hour before scooping into twelve balls. They'll keep in the fridge for up to two weeks.

#156 Banana Fat Bomb

Serves: 12

Time: 1 Hour 10 Minutes

Calories: 134

Protein: 3 Grams

Fat: 12 Grams

Net Carbs: 1 Gram

Ingredients:

- ¾ Cup Heavy Whipping Cream
- 6 Drops Liquid Stevia
- 1 Tablespoon Banana Extract, Pure
- 1 ¼ Cups Cream Cheese, Room Temperature

Directions:

1. Get out a baking sheet and line it with parchment paper, and then get out a bowl.
2. In your bowl beat together your heavy cream, cream cheese, stevia and banana extract. It should become thick and smooth, so you should beat it for about five minutes.
3. Spoon this mixture into mounds on your baking sheet, refrigerating until firm, which will take an hour.

#157 Pumpkin Spice Bomb

Serves: 16

Time: 1 Hour 10 Minutes

Calories: 87

Protein: 1 Gram

Fat: 9 Grams

Net Carbs: 1 Gram

Ingredients:

- 4 Drops Liquid Stevia
- 3 Tablespoons Almond, Chopped
- 1/3 Cup Pure Pumpkin Puree
- ½ Cup Cream Cheese, Room Temperature
- ½ Cup Butter, Room Temperature
- ¼ Teaspoon Nutmeg
- ½ Teaspoon Cinnamon

Directions:

1. Get out an eight by eight inch pan, lining it with parchment paper.
2. Get out a bowl, and whisk your cream cheese and butter together.
3. Add in your pumpkin puree, whisking again until it's well blended.
4. Stir in your cinnamon, stevia, nutmeg and almonds next.
5. Spoon this mixture into the pan, and then freeze for an hour.
6. Slice into sixteen pieces.

#158 Blueberry Bombs

Serves: 12

Time: 3 Hours 10 Minutes

Calories: 115

Protein: 1 Gram

Fat: 12 Grams

Net Carbs: 1 Gram

Ingredients:

- ½ Cup Coconut Oil, Room Temperature
- ½ Cup Cream Cheese, Room Temperature
- ½ Cup Blueberries, Mashed
- 6 Drops Liquid Stevia
- Pinch Ground Nutmeg

Directions:

1. Get out mini muffin tins, and then line it with paper liners.
2. In a bowl, mix your coconut oil and cream cheese until blended, and then stir in your stevia, nutmeg and blueberries. Make sure its mixed well, and then divide it between your muffin cups.
3. Freeze for three hours so it sets.

#159 Spiced Chocolate Bombs

Serves: 12

Time: 30 Minutes

Calories: 117

Protein: 2 Grams

Fat: 12 Grams

Net Carbs: 2 Grams

Ingredients:

- 3 Drops Liquid Stevia
- ¾ Cup Coconut Oil
- ¼ Cup Cocoa Powder
- 1/8 Teaspoon Chili Powder
- ¼ Cup Almond Butter

Directions:

1. Pull out a mini muffin tin, and then add paper liners.
2. Get out a saucepan, and then put it over low heat, adding in your cocoa powder, almond butter, coconut oil, stevia, and chili powder. Make sure it's heated all the way through and blended well.
3. Spoon this mixture into your muffin cups, and allow it to firm in the fridge for fifteen minutes. Store in the freezer until you're ready to serve them.

#160 Almond Butter Fudge

Serves: 36

Time: 2 Hours 10 Minutes

Calories: 204

Protein: 3 Grams

Fat: 22 Grams

Net Carbs: 2 Grams

Ingredients:

- 1 Cup Coconut Oil, Room Temperature
- 1 Cup Almond Butter
- 10 Drops Liquid Stevia
- Pinch Sea Salt
- ¼ Cup Heavy Whipping Cream

Directions:

1. Line a six by six inch baking dish using parchment paper before placing it to the side.
2. Whisk your coconut oil, almond butter, heavy cream, stevia and salt together until smooth, spooning the mixture into your baking dish. Smooth it out with your spatula, and then refrigerate for two hours so it your fudge can firm.
3. Cut into thirty-six pieces, and freeze until ready to serve.

#161 Coconut & Chocolate Candies

Serves: 16

Protein: 45 Minutes

Calories: 43

Protein: 1 Gram

Fat: 5 Grams

Net Carbs: 1 Gram

Ingredients:

- 4 Drops Liquid Stevia
- ¼ Cup Coconut, Shredded & Unsweetened
- 1/3 Cup Coconut Oil
- ¼ Cup Cocoa Powder, Unsweetened
- Pinch Sea Salt

Directions:

1. Get out a six by six inch pan, and line it with parchment paper.
2. Put a saucepan over low heat, adding in your cocoa, stevia, salt, and coconut toil. Heat together for three minutes and stir until well combined.
3. Stir in the coconut, pressing this mixture into your baking dish.
4. Refrigerate for a half hour, and then cut it into sixteen pieces.

#162 Raspberry Cheesecakes

Serves: 12

Time: 40 Minutes

Calories: 176

Protein: 6 Grams

Fat: 18 Grams

Net Carbs: 2 Grams

Ingredients:

- ½ Cup Cream Cheese, Room Temperature
- 2/3 Cup Coconut Oil, Melted
- 6 Eggs
- 3 Tablespoons Granulated Sweetener
- ½ Teaspoon Baking Powder
- ¾ Cup Raspberries
- 1 Teaspoon Vanilla Extract, Pure & Alcohol Free

Directions:

1. Start by heating your oven to 35, and then line an eight by eight in baking dish using parchment paper.
2. Get out a bowl and mix together your cream cheese and coconut oil, beating until smooth.
3. Beat your eggs, and then scrape down the sides of your bowl at least once.
4. Beat in your vanilla, baking powder and sweetener until its smooth.
5. Spoon the mixture into a baking dish, and scatter your raspberries across the top.

6. Bake until firm which should take twenty-five to thirty minutes.

7. Allow it to cool before slicing into twelve slices.

#163 Almond & Vanilla Pops

Serves: 8

Time: 4 Hours 15 Minutes

Calories: 166

Protein: 3 Grams

Fat: 15 Grams

Net Carbs: 2 Grams

Ingredients:

- 2 Cups Almond Milk
- 1 Cup Heavy Whipping Cream
- 1 Vanilla Bean, Halved
- 1 Cup Coconut, Shredded & Unsweetened

Directions:

1. Put a saucepan over medium heat, adding in your heavy cream, vanilla bean and almond milk, letting it simmer before reducing it to low. Continue to simmer for another five minutes, and then remove it from heat. Allow it to cool, and then take out your vanilla bean. Scrape the seeds back into the liquid.
2. Stir in your coconut, and then divide it between your molds.
3. Freeze it for four hours.

Conclusion

Now you know everything you need to know in order to get started with your meal prepping today! Make sure that your kitchen is fully stocked and ready before you get started. Remember that containers are important to keeping your food safe to eat and easy to take on the go. Just make sure that you plan out what meals you want to cook in advance to keep a healthy variety of meals that will last you through breakfast to dessert every day of the week. The ketogenic diet can be stressful, but with meal prepping, it's easier to stick to your diet and weight loss goals.

9 781725 764200